SUN SEEKERS
THE CURE OF CALIFORNIA

Lyra Kilston

ATELIER ÉDITIONS

3

One bright January morning I was driving to the desert to visit an archive when I saw a freeway exit sign for Beaumont, a small town over an hour east of Los Angeles. The name triggered a recollection so I made a detour. I wended through a broad valley south of the dry San Bernardino Mountains, past horse pastures, beige tract housing, and mobile homes.

When I came to the Highland Springs Resort I turned up a driveway splitting an orchard of silvery olive trees. I parked and began exploring the quiet grounds. Small white cottages that once housed patients fringed a meandering path, tucked between oak trees, cacti, and flowering bushes. Birds darted between sun and shade; orange butterflies eddied in the warm air.

5

I peered through a padlocked gate at the mineral baths and a bathhouse with a rocky, arched facade. The pool was empty, a layer of dark leaves at its bottom.

Several months earlier, while researching an obscure German dietician named Arnold Ehret for this book, I was scrolling through digitized pages of newspapers nearly a century old. One announced a new health resort in Beaumont based on Ehret's principles. When I had looked up the resort, I was amazed to discover it still existed. I filed this fact away and forgot all about it until I saw the sign.

In the late 1920s, two brothers, Fred and Will Hirsch, ardent devotees of Ehret's, purchased 320 acres with a stagecoach-era hotel for the resort. The brothers first met Ehret about a decade earlier in Los Angeles, where the German emigrant gave frequent public lectures on his theories of natural health. Ehret's regimen was strict: no caffeine, alcohol, meat, or processed foods, daily exercise, sun baths, and regular bouts of fasting to clear the body of toxic, disease-causing matter. This embrace of nature's gifts, he believed, could cure all bodily ills—from cancer to the pain of childbirth to aging. In the photographs included in his slim, maniacal books, Ehret's face is chiseled, with a mustache like two arrows and eyes burning with intensity (or hunger). A sketch made of him after a 49-day fast shows the peaceful visage of an enlightened, long-haired messiah.

Fred Hirsch, who had long suffered from an incurable illness, decided to follow Ehret's instructions to fast for 30 days and whittle his diet down to only fruit and vegetables. According to Fred himself, he was miraculously cured. Converted, he devoted himself to helping Ehret translate, publish, and publicize his books. He became his friend and partner and was present at his untimely death in 1922.

6

In 1928, Fred and his brother opened the first and only 'Ehretist' resort in America, in the small town of Beaumont. It attracted Ehret's devotees as well as curious health seekers. Sometimes called 'The Last Resort', it drew hundreds of patients who, like Fred Hirsch, had exhausted all other methods of recovery. A fruit orchard and a large garden supplied the vegetarian dining room, while the mineral springs were claimed to cure everything from neuritis to rheumatism. However, despite the brothers' fidelity to their deceased health guru, the strict Ehretist phase was short-lived. The rustic property has changed hands and uses several times in the intervening years: to a summer camp for affluent Jewish families, then a ranch, and recently a farm, hotel, and wedding venue.

As I wandered around the resort looking for vestiges of the 1920s, I met a friendly woman who worked there. She was inside one of the original modest cottages; a ring of them had been turned into gift shops offering farm products such as olive oil, kombucha, and lavender. She explained that the property would soon be relaunched as a wellness center based on ecological education, sustainability, and a farm-to-table lifestyle. There would be farm camps for children and old-fashioned craft workshops for adults, teaching skills like knitting and baking bread. She noted that there was some sourdough in the oven right now, if I had time to wait.

The resort's rebirth seemed like a continuation of Ehret's heal-by-nature dogma updated for a new century. In the course of our conversation the woman paused and asked if I had heard about the health benefits of fermented foods. "Of course," I answered, settling into stereotype, "I live in L.A.!" "I'm not sure if you know all the facts," she said, becoming more serious, "but fermented foods will *radically* improve pretty much every aspect of your health." I looked at her

7

quizzically. I asked if she had heard of Arnold Ehret, whose philosophy had long ago graced the acreage we stood on. She had not.

Ehret is no household name. In fact, to his dismay, it never was. But he was part of a wave of remarkable, eccentric health pioneers in the region whose names have been almost lost to history. (Almost, but not quite: Steve Jobs, for instance, discovered Ehret's work in the early 1970s, in Oregon, and dabbled in fasting and a raw-fruit diet.) I learned about Ehret while digging into the same source that launched this book: a beguiling black-and-white photograph showing a group of bearded, long-haired men holding wedges of watermelon. Some were bare-chested or wore white sarongs. Standard California hippies—except the photo was from the 1940s. Who were these men? What I eventually uncovered is part of the fascinating history of how California became a center for healthy, natural living.

Health fads thrive on collective amnesia: they must always be new, a discovery, a miracle. A new way to eat, a new way to live, and to live longer. Even when linked to ancient ways of life, like today's slow- or raw-food movements, meditation, or the Paleo diet, the practices appear fresh to each convert. There is a perpetual cycle of zealous rediscovery—whole grains, fruit juice, fermentation—it's the latest thing and will change your life.

"I thought California would be different," wrote Raymond Pettibon, the artist, in a drawing in 1989. His phrase echoes backward and forward in time. Newcomers still arrive expecting to be alchemized— thinking life will be different, that they themselves will be different. Lay straw under this constant, coastal sun and watch it harden into gold. California's dense layers of mythology and cliché endure for better or worse, continually resurrected by new seekers grasping at that steady, sun-gilded mirage.

Even before the state was incorporated in 1850, and before flakes of gold were discovered in a cold river two years earlier, California's myth-making machinery was cranking up to unspool a bright streak of promise. Generations sought freedom, wilderness, prosperity, a rupture from the old ways, a new beginning. And following behind, swiftly dismantling each fable, came a counter-parade, a chorus of brilliantly acerbic critics pointing toward apocalypse. Myth-makers, myth-breakers: the pendulum swings.

What follows is an account of a myth whose history has received less fanfare than the well-known stories of local gold—gleaming veins in the rocks, then celluloid, then silicon—the myth of California as a cure in itself. A giant natural sanatorium for the revival of the body and the self. Its seekers were many—this myth of health sparked its own, lesser known, rush in the last quarter of the nineteenth century. They sought the auric, perpetual sunshine that enriches swaths of bare skin, fortifies vegetation and pours through broad windows, bringing the outdoors inside. They sought both physical health and something more holistic and abstract, a source of vitality far from the poisons of civilization. A wellspring reclaimed; a return to nature. Some found what they were looking for.

Although its influence has oscillated, this health rush has never waned. It still marks the region's culture, reputation, and physical landscape in the constant flood of diet, wellness, and fitness trends; in strange-smelling tinctures lining grocery store shelves or in empty mineral baths now filled with leaves. This book tells the stories of a few of the seekers who came to the wilder edge of this continent in pursuit of various interpretations of 'health'—what they found, how they lived, and which forces propelled them here.

9

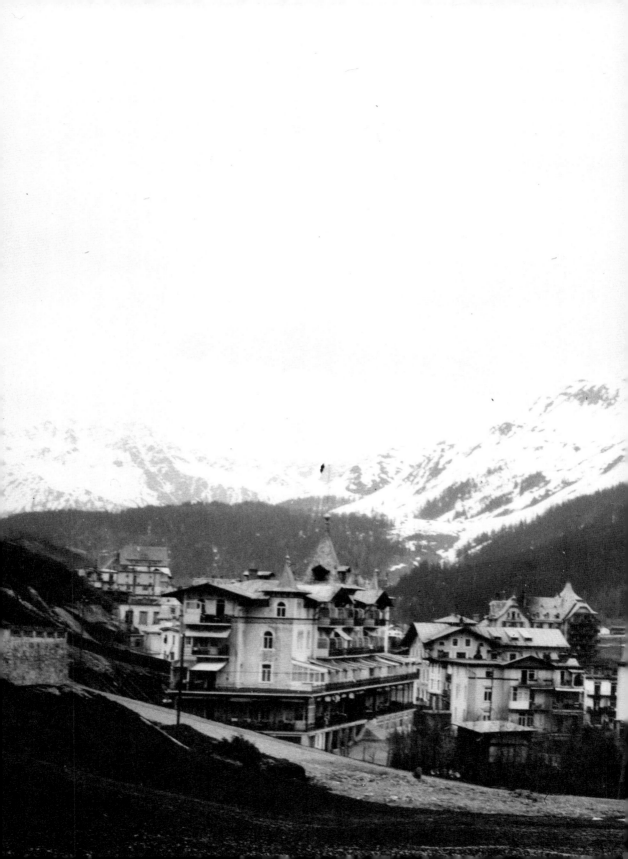

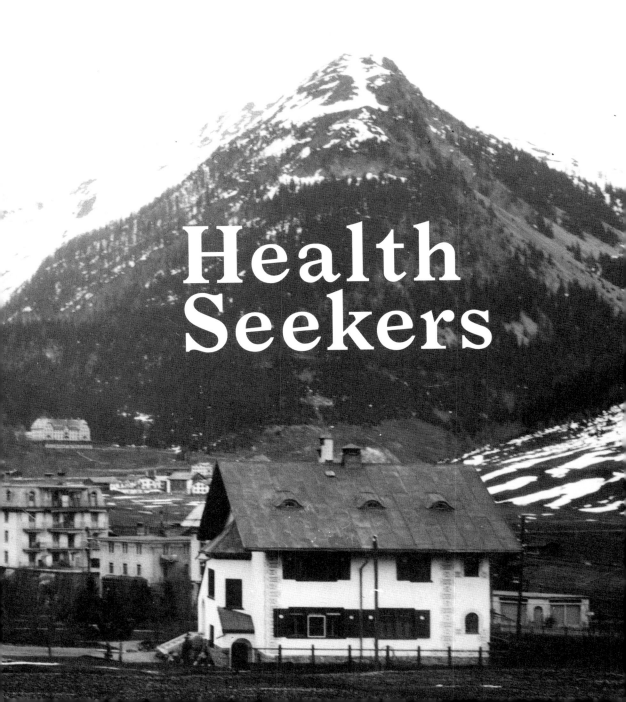

Health
Seekers

"Climate is to a country what temperament is to a man—Fate."

Helen Hunt Jackson

previous page — View of Davos Sanatorium, Switzerland, circa 1920.

In the spring of 1602, Basque merchant Sebastián Vizcaíno was sent on a mission to map the California coast for Spain. Several months later, he and his crew docked in a placid bay he named San Diego and some of them went ashore to explore the foreign terrain. There they encountered an astonishing woman who looked "more than one hundred and fifty years old."

As Vizcaino's journal recounts, the men crossed the sandy beach and were met by a large group of native people armed with bows and arrows. Emerging from the group was the wrinkled, elderly woman, who approached the sailors as an envoy. She was frightened of the pale-skinned, strangely dressed intruders and wept as she walked. The Spaniards, in turn, were shocked by her extremely aged appearance. Her name went unrecorded, but her deeply creased belly was described as looking "like a blacksmith's bellows." The sailors offered her beads and something to eat to show their peaceable aims. Tensions broke and civil relations between the two cultures were established, at least for the day.

The story of this impossibly long-lived woman may be one of the earliest sources of one of Southern California's most enduring myths: the land's ability to enhance longevity.

Centuries passed without much outside interest in the region beyond that of Spanish colonizers. But in the mid-nineteenth century a trickle of immigration became a flood, transforming the newly incorporated state. Gold was one lure. Another was the opportunity to explore and document this wild land, which was perceived as new and empty. Adventurers wrote in rapturous detail of grapes and citrus fruit bursting from the rich soil, tranquil weather patterns, and the varied landscape of mountains, deserts, forests, and ocean. The mysteriously long lifespans of the native elders were also noted repeatedly, adding a supernatural air to the already intriguing land.

HEALTH SEEKERS

Doctors, too, fed into the lore. "The climate is so healthy that illness is rarely found and one sees many persons who have reached an age of over a hundred years," wrote Dr. J. Praslow, who had come to California from Germany in 1849 to practice medicine. During his travels around the state by horse, foot, and wagon, he saw "people here who were from 100 to 115 years old and who were still very active." Praslow was one of the first medically trained observers to link California's geography and climate to its residents' longevity, and he set out to make a comprehensive "medico-geographical" study. He concluded from his records of daily temperature, sun exposure, and agriculture that excellent health could be expected for incoming Pacific Coast settlers.

A few years later, British-American physician Dr. James Blake reported similar findings in the *American Journal of the Medical Sciences*:

"I am but expressing my candid opinion when I state, that I believe California will be found more conducive to the highest physical and intellectual development of the Anglo-Saxon race, than any other part of the globe. There is not a day in the year in which the powers of the mind or of the body are enervated by heat or numbed by cold. And when the agricultural resources of the country shall become developed, and the swamp lands reclaimed and brought under cultivation, I believe that every external influence, detrimental to the preservation of health, will be reduced to a minimum."

Dr. Peter Charles Remondino, an Italian-born physician who co-founded San Diego's first private hospital, described the locale in a medical journal as a "paradise of old age." He believed that the region was capable of "setting back, so to speak, the march of our age for a generation or more." Furthermore, he claimed that the extended lifespan of the native people could be achieved by Caucasian settlers, leading them to new heights of physical and mental perfection.

The source of this radiant health was proclaimed to be purely climatic, never genetic or cultural. (Indeed, the same climate that was thought to improve Anglo settlers was seen as causing the indigenous populations to become idle and morally lax.) It was the land, the weather, the *place*, that enabled such long lifespans. One only needed to relocate to reap its benefits.

Connecting health to locale is often traced back to Hippocrates, who wrote the treatise *On Airs, Waters, and Places* around the fifth century BCE. It prescribed the ideal orientation of winds, water sources, seasons, and sun exposure for a person to pursue a modest diet and regular exercise. The influence of his theory fluctuated over the centuries but gained immense sway in Europe and the United States in the mid-to-late nineteenth century as illnesses soared and doctors often proved helpless.

By 1860, the notion that health was dependent on place was widely accepted. Eastern American cities, with their humidity, long wet winters, and dense populations, augured inescapable disease. Doctors prescribed journeys to the West or Southwest for climatotherapy, citing the "radically curative and reinvigorating influences" of fresh dry air, ample sunshine, and new scenery.

Meanwhile, California's climate cure was exalted in newspaper advertisements, handbooks, and travel guides. Readers in the Midwest and on both sides of the Atlantic were told of constant sunshine and near-instantaneous health recoveries. (One journalist in Pasadena, a town east of Los Angeles, satirized the deluge of boastful miracle-cure testimonies by stating, "When I left home I had but one lung and it almost gone... I have been two weeks in Pasadena [and now] have three lungs.")

15

California was garlanded with romantic monikers and compared to salubrious sites abroad: "The Better Italy," "The Land of Sunshine," "The New Palestine," and "A Geographical Pleiades," among others. A magazine editorial by the president of the San Diego Chamber of Commerce displays the soapbox tone typical of the time:

"What is the foundation of the prosperity of Southern California?" The answer lies in the single word—climate. Climate is the underlying basis upon which the present is established and the future assured. "But," says the caviler [sic], sneeringly, "one can't live on climate." That is the mistake. One can live on climate; and throughout the length and breadth of Southern California, we all do."

Aided by the new transcontinental railroad, tens of thousands of people began to head west, permanently transforming the region. About a quarter of them came because of illness and were known as "health seekers." Historian John E. Baur, noting the newcomers' belief that locale alone could replace medical care, facetiously suggested a nickname for the area: "Dr. Southern California." The promises of miraculous recovery were inflated, certainly, and their wide acceptance may appear naive. But many desperately ill Americans, having tried every other known cure, pinned their last hopes on this arid, sun-drenched 'doctor.'

"TB [tuberculosis] is often imagined as a disease of poverty and deprivation—of thin garments, thin bodies, unheated rooms, poor hygiene, inadequate food... There was a notion that TB was a wet disease, a disease of humid and dank cities. The inside of the body became damp ('moisture in the lungs' was a favored locution) and had to be dried out. Doctors advised travel to high, dry places—the mountains, the desert."
— Susan Sontag, *Illness as Metaphor*

The nineteenth century witnessed a grim march of epidemic diseases without remedy. Tuberculosis was the most widespread. It was the leading cause of death in Europe and the United States, where an estimated 70 to 90 percent of the urban population was infected and eight in ten of those who ultimately contracted the disease died.

Known as 'consumption' and the 'white plague,' tuberculosis could kill rapidly, or recede and return many years later. It was believed to be hereditary, but inflamed by poor living and working conditions. In 1882 it was discovered to be contagious, but no cure was found for nearly seventy years. Contagion was so acute that infection could occur just by breathing near an invalid; overcrowded urban areas were the most devastated, and women were more often afflicted than men due to the constraints of their indoor lives.

Medical practice often caused more harm than healing. Purging and blistering were employed, and doses of addictive laudanum and poisonous mercury were prescribed, all of which sapped the little strength patients had left. For much of that century, doctors believed the Medieval theory that sickness was frequently induced by 'miasma'—bad or poisonous vapors arising from decomposing matter. (Some believed that a mere breath of miasmatic air, whether it drifted from a sewage-filled city river or radiated from steaming jungles in the tropics, caused the body to begin to decompose and ferment.)

At the same time, urban populations were growing exponentially, while cities' antiquated systems of plumbing, sewage, and trash collection—not to mention cemeteries—struggled unsuccessfully to keep pace. In New York City a state legislative committee described the condition of tenements in the late 1850s:

"The dim, undrained courts oozing with pollution; the dark, narrow stairways, decayed with age, reeking with filth, over-run with vermin; the rotted floors, ceilings begrimed, and often too low to permit you to stand upright..."

Across the ocean, London held up a bleak mirror. In the East End, known as 'darkest London,' novelist Arthur Morrison described the slum floridly:

"Black and noisome, the road sticky with slime, and palsied houses, rotten from chimney to cellar... Dark, silent, uneasy shadows passing and crossing—human vermin in this reek-ing sink, like goblin exhalations from all that is noxious around."

Wood and coal burning, and pollution from the rapidly proliferating factories, plunged cities into a blurry haze of soot. The streets ran with animal waste, and cesspools emptied into rivers. Industrial laborers (including children) worked without ventilation or other safety standards, twelve hours a day, six days a week. The homes of the urban working classes were often dim and damp. Rooms were typically stuffed with fussy germ-harboring carpets, wallpaper, and thick curtains. Windows were kept closed against drafts, while densely built housing blocked sunlight. Poor health was worsened by the typical diet, which included very little fresh produce. (Some doctors had blamed the mid-century cholera epidemic on the consumption of vegetables, banning their sale for a time.) As one medical researcher complained, for many in England the daily fare was solely "tea and bread, bread and tea." Lack of regular bathing and hygiene also took its toll. The climate, the home, and the body all bred illness.

The antidote to this threatening urban existence, rife with contagion and disease, beckoned. *The mountains, the desert.* Southern California had both—for those who could afford to get there. The sky was cloudless, nights cool, days brilliant, nature abundant. No slums or industry yet existed to stain the air. An official (and certainly biased) state health report of 1870 proclaimed California the "Sanatorium of the World."

Leaflet Number 6. (For Children.)
California Association for the Study and Prevention of Tuberculosis.

The Tuberculosis [Consumption] Problem.*
WHAT CHILDREN SHOULD KNOW ABOUT IT.

The Useful Citizens of a Nation.

Healthy citizens are able to do their work better than sick citizens. Healthy citizens are, on that account, worth more to a country. That is why sickness causing much death is a matter of public concern.

A Disease That Causes Much Unnecessary Sickness and Death.

Tuberculosis of the lungs or consumption causes every year the death of almost two hundred thousand citizens in the United States. Nearly all of these persons are past the age of fifteen.

The money loss from these deaths has been calculated to be every year more than three hundred million dollars for the United States alone!

For these reasons all children should resolve to learn about this disease and aid in its prevention.

Tuberculosis Is Not Inherited.

It is true that tuberculosis often "runs in families," but that does not mean that the disease is "inherited." It simply means that the person who first had the disease did not take sufficient care to prevent other members of the family from taking the disease.

The Causes of Tuberculosis.

The real cause of tuberculosis is a little plant, called a germ, which gets into the body and feeds on the lungs like a parasite.

An unhealthy body helps the germ to get a foothold and start the disease. A healthy body is usually able to kill the germ before it does much mischief. So that to get tuberculosis a certain germ must get into an unhealthy body.

How the Germ Is Spread About.

A person with tuberculosis usually has a cough. With a cough, such a person often brings up stuff from the lungs called sputum. This sputum of a single consumptive in a single day may contain millions and millions of the germs.

When this sputum dries, the germs are scattered far and wide with the dust, getting on the food we eat, the things we handle and in the air we breathe.

How to Kill the Germ.

The best way is to always destroy the sputum that is coughed up. If the sputum is coughed into paper cups or napkins these can be burned and the germs destroyed.

After the sputum has dried to dust, to kill all the germs is almost impossible.

How People Get Weak Bodies.

People get weak bodies because some persons are born weak, but most people become weak after sickness like measles or grippe, or they may become weak because they work or study too hard, or because they have not sufficient food or eat improper food, or because they breathe impure air, or because they have bad habits.

How to Prevent Tuberculosis.

First, keep the germ from getting into the bodies of people, particularly of persons whose health is not good.

This can be done by having persons with tuberculosis always destroy their sputum as directed. Spitting on the floor or ground or coughing into people's faces should also be avoided.

Second, all persons should be in good health. To be so, pure air must be constantly breathed, night time as well as day time; nourishing food must be eaten and the proper amounts of rest and exercise taken.

The Cure of Tuberculosis.

Tuberculosis is cured by making the body healthy. Pure air, good food and rest, with a competent physician to watch the patient, will do this better than any medicine.

WRITTEN BY GEORGE H. KRESS.

*This is Educational Leaflet number 6 (For Children) issued by the California Association for the Study and Prevention of Tuberculosis. Single copies, one cent each. Larger lots, prices on application. Office of the Association, 240 Bradbury Bldg., Los Angeles, Cal.

Copies of this and other literature on prevention and cure sent gratis on application.

Other Anti-Tuberculosis Societies are given permission to republish these leaflets, on condition that credit is given to the California Association for the Study and Prevention of Tuberculosis.

THE STORY OF TUBERCULOSIS—BRIEFLY TOLD IN PICTURES.

HOW THE GERMS OF CONSUMPTION ARE CARRIED FROM THE SICK TO THE WELL

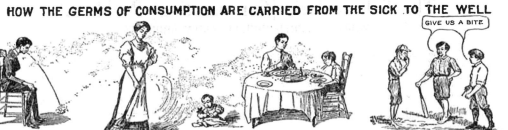

CONSUMPTIVE SPITTING ON FLOOR. FLIES FEEDING ON IT, CARRY THE GERMS OF THE DISEASE TO FOOD.

THE SPIT DRIES AND CARELESS SWEEPING, DUSTING OR DRAUGHTS CAUSE THE GERMS TO FLOAT IN THE AIR.

THE GERMS MAY ENTER THE BODIES OF CHILDREN PLAYING ON THE FLOOR, THROUGH SORES OR WOUNDS.

OTHERS MAY GET THE DISEASE BY BREATHING OR SWALLOWING THE GERMS. SPRAY GIVEN OFF IN SNEEZING OR COUGHING, CONTAINS GERMS IN A MOIST AND ACTIVE STATE.

PUTTING FOOD, MONEY, PENCILS ETC. INTO THE MOUTH AFTER A CONSUMPTIVE HAS POISONED THEM WITH HIS SPIT.

NEW YORK STATE DEPARTMENT OF HEALTH.

CONSUMPTIONS ALLIES—AVOID THEM AND YOU ARE SAFEGUARDING AGAINST THE DISEASE

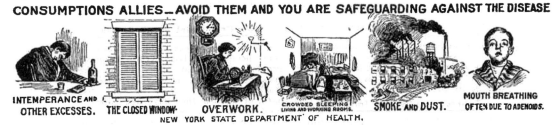

INTEMPERANCE AND OTHER EXCESSES.

THE CLOSED WINDOW.

OVERWORK.

CROWDED SLEEPING LIVING AND WORKING ROOMS.

SMOKE AND DUST.

MOUTH BREATHING OFTEN DUE TO ADENOIDS.

NEW YORK STATE DEPARTMENT OF HEALTH.

IN CASE OF CONSUMPTION, LOOK TO THESE FOR CURE

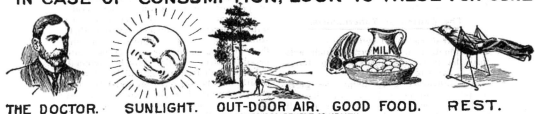

THE DOCTOR. SUNLIGHT. OUT-DOOR AIR. GOOD FOOD. REST.

NEW YORK STATE DEPARTMENT OF HEALTH.

A CAREFUL CONSUMPTIVE,—NOT DANGEROUS TO LIVE WITH,

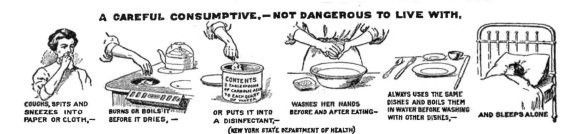

COUGHS, SPITS AND SNEEZES INTO PAPER OR CLOTH,—

BURNS OR BOILS IT BEFORE IT DRIES, —

OR PUTS IT INTO A DISINFECTANT,—

WASHES HER HANDS BEFORE AND AFTER EATING—

ALWAYS USES THE SAME DISHES AND BOILS THEM IN WATER BEFORE WASHING WITH OTHER DISHES,—

AND SLEEPS ALONE

(NEW YORK STATE DEPARTMENT OF HEALTH)

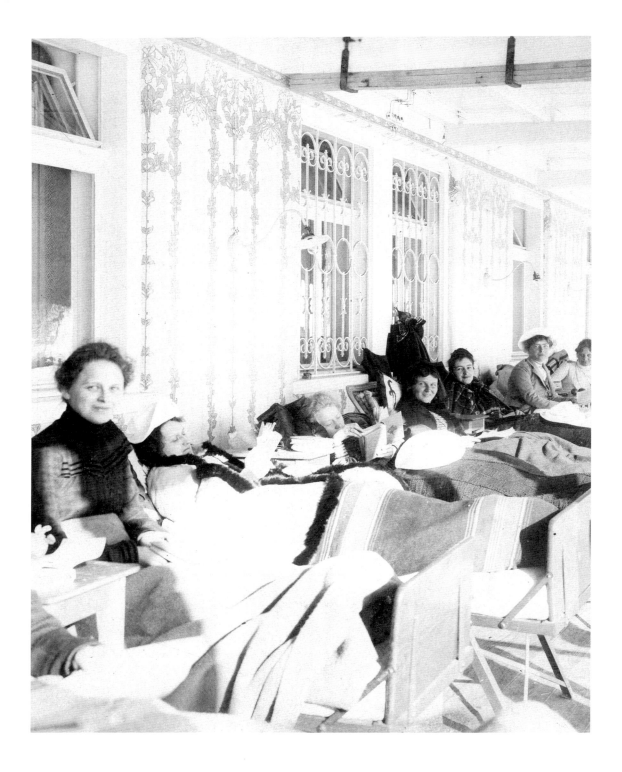

22

previous page — **California Society for Prevention of Tuberculosis pamphlet, 1908.**
above — **Patients take in the sun at a spa hotel, Davos, Switzerland, circa 1903.**

In Southern California, early health seekers embraced the sunshine, fresh air, and opportunity to sleep outdoors. To reap the benefits of particular micro-climates, they often lived somewhat nomadically, circulating among various hotels, boarding houses, or crudely erected tent cities. One family traveled for months by horse-drawn house-wagon, wandering in search of the warmest and driest places. Another family pitched a carpet over a tree branch and lived beneath its peaked shelter for six weeks. An ill Massa-chusetts man wandered the bucolic Ojai Valley with a cow, subsisting only on its raw milk until he claimed a miraculous recovery.

Such makeshift regimens, reliant on climactic cures, were also practiced in the warmer parts of Europe. But a more formalized health infrastructure was being developed there, blending the efficiency of a hospital with the comforts of a hotel, and sited well outside of cities. A pastoral setting was crucial, reflecting the popular belief in the curative powers of nature. This particular medical philosophy became known as naturopathy, a holistic approach that focused on preventative care, centering on medicines made from plants and the gentler cures of a healthy diet, sunlight, fresh air, and water.

One of the first known conventionally trained doc-tors to use a naturopathic approach for tuberculosis was George Bodington. An English country doctor who had apprenticed to a surgeon and earned an apothecary license, Bodington purchased a private mental asylum outside of Birmingham to treat patients with his "open-air" cure sometime before 1833. In 1840 he published his treatise, *On the Treatment and Cure of Pulmonary Tuberculosis*, which condemned the local medical methods of blistering, starvation, and confinement in a closed room, and advocated instead for fresh air, gentle exercise, and a varied diet. He also called for hospitals serving the poor to offer such amenities. Unfortunately, his ideas were considered crude and offensive by the medical establishment, and he was loudly condemned in the leading medical journal *The Lancet*. Discouraged, he abandoned his research and spent the rest of his career treating mental illness instead. When Bodington died, in 1882, his pioneering methods had become widely practiced; in its obituary *The Lancet* offered a tardy apology and hailed the doctor's remarkable foresight.

Soon after Bodington published his treatise, however, similar ideas were finding fertile ground to the east. In Görbersdorf, a village tucked into a pristine valley near what is now the Polish-Czech border, hydropathic physician Countess Marie von Colomb opened a water-cure clinic, following the lead of her teacher, the famous self-taught Silesian peasant Vincenz Priessnitz, a.k.a. the "father of hydrotherapy." Görbersdorf, surrounded by the lushly forested slopes of the Stone Mountains, offered clean air and fresh water, and like Priessnitz's popular clinic, was at high altitude.[1]

Colomb's clinic prescribed a regimen of wet compresses, drinking copious amounts of spring water, several cold showers and baths daily, vigorous hikes, and sleeping with windows open in all seasons. Pleased with the clinic's progress and its tranquil setting, she invited her brother-in-law, Dr. Hermann Brehmer, to visit. A botanist-turned physician, Brehmer was also in search of a healthful locale to begin receiving patients. His medical research on the treatment of tuberculosis was centered on the theory of an "immune place." After touring the valley and seeing Colomb's clinic, he agreed that the location might offer the elusive immunity he sought.

Launching his practice in Görbersdorf, Brehmer began to treat a small number of consumptive patients. His system included water treatments and hiking (or "methodical hill-climbing" as he called it) as well as a diet of milk, fatty foods, vegetables, and a nightcap of cognac. In time he was able to acquire a large piece of land and undertake the construction of an imposing, thick-walled institution he called a *Heilanstalt*, or "healing place." (Some accounts credit Colomb as having co-founded it with Brehmer.) It opened in the late 1850s, and as word spread of this new type of tuberculosis treatment, and its magnificent facility and location, the Heilanstalt grew, over time, to house several hundred patients.

Fusing the grandeur of towering Gothic architecture with elements of a homey alpine chalet, Brehmer's sanatorium (as it would be called) offered the amenities required for an extended stay. It boasted a medical laboratory, a meteorological observatory, a vast library, men's and women's parlors, dining rooms, bedrooms with windows meant to remain ajar, two indoor gardens and its own dairy—under strict hygienic supervision. No carpeting was permitted (a fibrous den of germs!), and air shafts and ventilators kept fresh air recycling. The sanatorium was surrounded by a vast forest laced with walking paths, which Brehmer 'prescribed' to his patients, matching various levels of exertion to their gradually improving strength. He believed that high-altitude exercise would strengthen the hearts of tubercular patients, which in turn would heal their lungs. This was not strictly true, but nonetheless his treatments did improve the health of many patients who arrived in the early stages of illness.

Brehmer's methods, and his synthesis of medical sci-

1. Priessnitz advocated for cold-water treatments, breaking from the established European spa traditions of seaside cures and visits to pungent mineral springs. His methods brought skepticism from many (local authorities often raided his clinic to examine his sponges for sorcery or hidden drugs), but were widely replicated and absorbed into other health regimens.

Priessnitz's methods were popularized in America via Dr. John Harvey Kellogg of the famed Battle Creek Sanitarium in Michigan, a Christian health resort founded in 1866 that embraced the natural forces of sunlight, water, and whole grains, but forbade pharmaceuticals, meat, alcohol, sex, and masturbation.

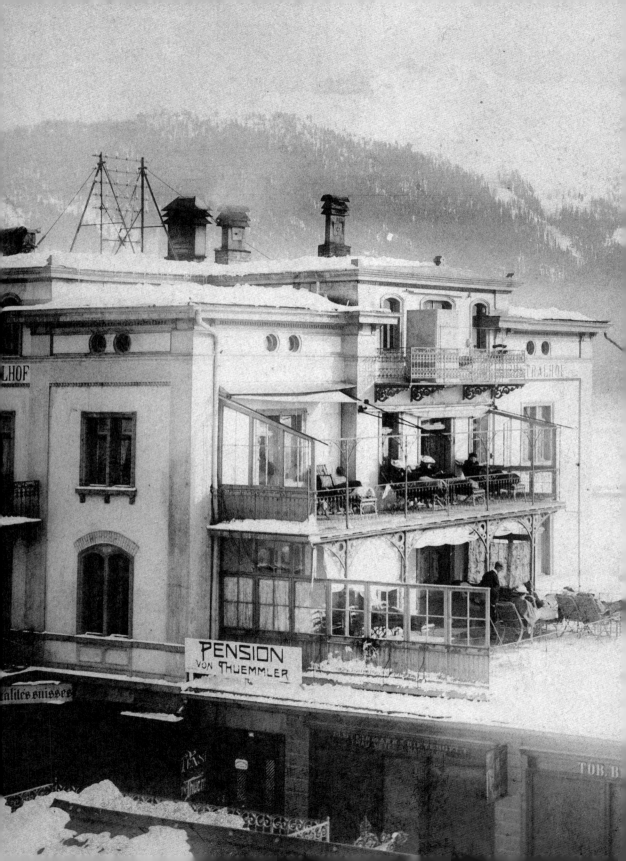

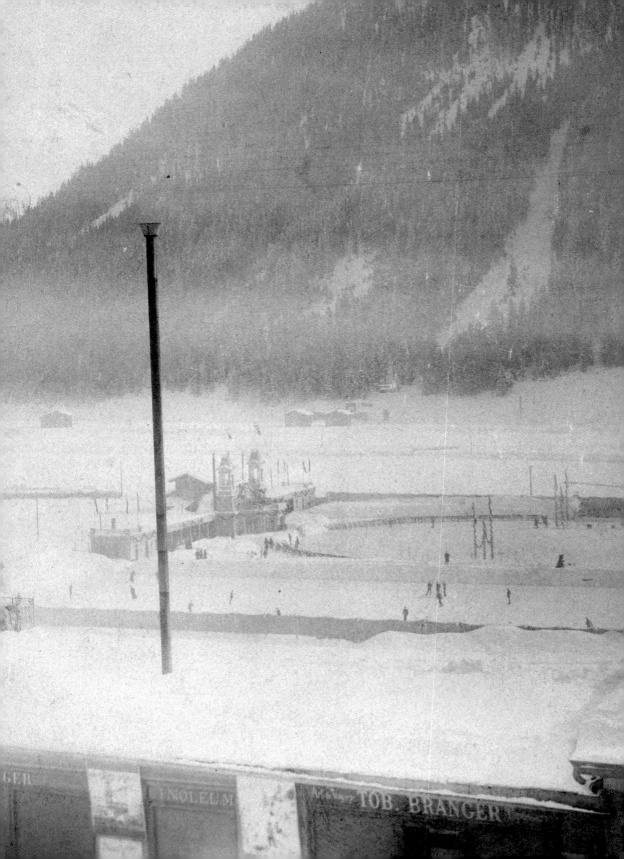

ence with the healing properties of a salubrious locale, sparked a sanatorium movement that spread across Europe.[2] The trend proliferated first in mountainous regions, where the sunlight was stronger and the air so clean it was said to taste like champagne. High-altitude villages like Görbersdorf and Davos, Switzerland, became famous health resorts, attracting patients who could afford the fees from across the continent.

Davos's renown began with Dr. Alexander Spengler, a German physician assigned to serve the mile-high farming village. Astride his horse with his doctor's bag in tow, Spengler visited patients in the snowbound valley and began to notice an intriguing lack of tuberculosis. Instead it was common, he observed, for locals to possess "a beautiful, symmetrical body, a bulging chest and a strong heart muscle," as well as impressive stamina for scaling steep mountain slopes without becoming breathless. Was it possible this, like Görbersdorf, was another immune place?

Spengler could soon put his hypothesis to the test. In the middle of the bleak winter of 1865, he received two frail German patients who had heard rumors of the illness-free valley. Exhausted from the nine-hour sleigh ride to reach Davos, the men were taken under Spengler's care. They followed the doctor's instructions, most importantly exposing themselves daily to the pure, bracing mountain air, and recovered after one season, spreading their triumphant story far and wide. Spengler, too, broadcast his victory to the medical community, and set about building a *Kurhaus* (cure-house). It possessed long, wide porches for outdoor rest, where patients lay on chaise longues for hours, imbibing sunlight and crisp air. His healing regimen was quite unique. He prescribed 'stabulation' (sleeping in cowsheds) so that patients would inhale the pungent vapors of the animals' urine; the taking of cold showers even when the spray would turn to ice; and massages with marmot fat—a rich liniment rendered from the

previous page — View of a spa hotel, with patients on balconies, Davos, Switzerland, circa 1903.

alpine rodent and believed to be both curative and easily absorbed.

Eventually, good rail connections helped Davos become one of Europe's most popular locations for health seekers. At first they came only in summer, but belief in the antiseptic benefits of the unsullied, frosty air soon brought them in droves, in winter as well, to wade thigh-deep through the snow and sleep with windows flung wide open. More sanatoriums opened to receive the ever-increasing flood of patients. Their architecture evoked the lavish, hotel-like model of Brehmer's in Görbersdorf, but enhanced the patients' exposure to sunlight and mountain air through south-facing windows, porches, and balconies. Frequently the rooms featured hygienic interiors, with linoleum flooring and disinfectable furniture. Dietary regimens varied, but each institution monitored its patients' meals closely and prescribed schedules of rest, promenades, hydrotherapy, and ceaseless exposure to fresh air. To ameliorate the isolation, and the constant shadow of death, familiar domestic distractions were offered. One account of an alpine sanatorium, in the 1892 edition of *The Illustrated American* journal, described patients "clothed in long flannel dresses, up to their necks in water in a common bath, where they remain for several hours together. Each bather had a small floating table before him, from which his book, newspaper, or coffee is enjoyed."

The salutary mystique of Davos was famously immortalized in Thomas Mann's novel *The Magic Mountain*, which follows the existential adventures of Hans Castorp, a young engineer who plans to spend only a few weeks visiting his cousin at one of the village's grand tuberculosis sanatoriums, but ends up

2. Sanatorium, or sanitarium, or sanitorium? The difference lies between Latin roots sanare (to heal, to cure), and sanitas (healthy, sane). The spelling varied by country, and sometimes even by doctor. With such similar roots, the results were often muddled. Here, 'sanatorium' is used to mean a nature-cure institution.

remaining as a patient in its suspended twilight for seven years. As Castorp approaches the institution for the first time, he sees "a long building, with a cupola and so many balconies that from a distance it looked porous, like a sponge." Once inside, "the walls gleamed with hard white enamel paint... the room looked restful and cheery, with practical white furniture, white washable walls, clean linoleum, and white linen curtains gaily embroidered in modern taste."[3] Here, Castorp falls under the spell of the clinic and the sublime Alps, where time slows and the outside world "down there" recedes.

The mountains of Europe were considered magical for a time, capable of saving lives by virtue of their bracing winds, tonic springs, and resin-scented air. The pathologist and historian Thomas Dormandy surmised that this notion of enchanted altitude likely "owed more to the lyric poetry of Goethe, the songs of Schubert, and the vision of moonlit forests and snow-capped mountain peaks by Caspar David Friedrich, than to scientific mumbo-jumbo about metabolic purification." Either way, even as sanatoriums emerged on the flatlands, the mountains retained an aura of purity and health that has never entirely faded.

Soon, 'taking the cure' at a sanatorium became entrenched in European culture, with its own customs, tools, and rituals. Or, it came to seem as normal as a reason can be to leave behind one's home and family for an unknown period of time.

right — View of Sokolowsko (known as Görbersdorf in German) Sanatorium, run by Dr. Brehmer.

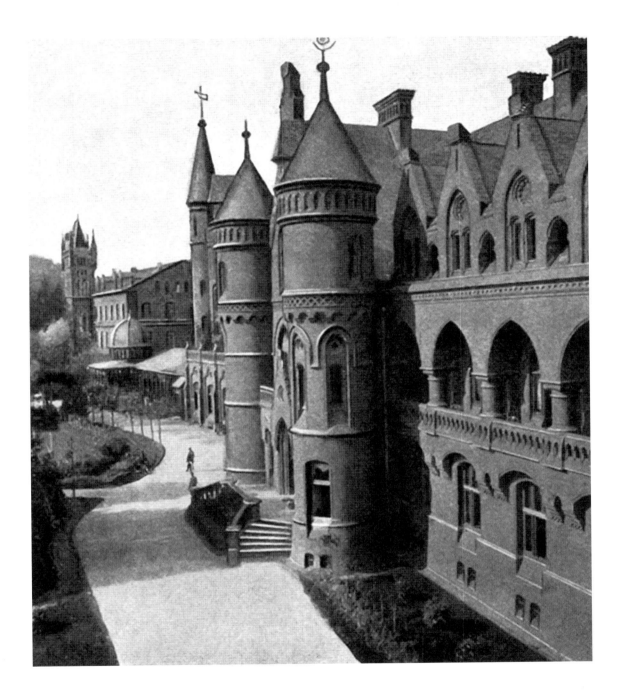

3. Thomas Mann had witnessed the Swiss
therapeutic lifestyle first-hand when he
visited his ailing wife, Katia, in Davos's
Waldsanatorium in 1912.

HEALTH SEEKERS

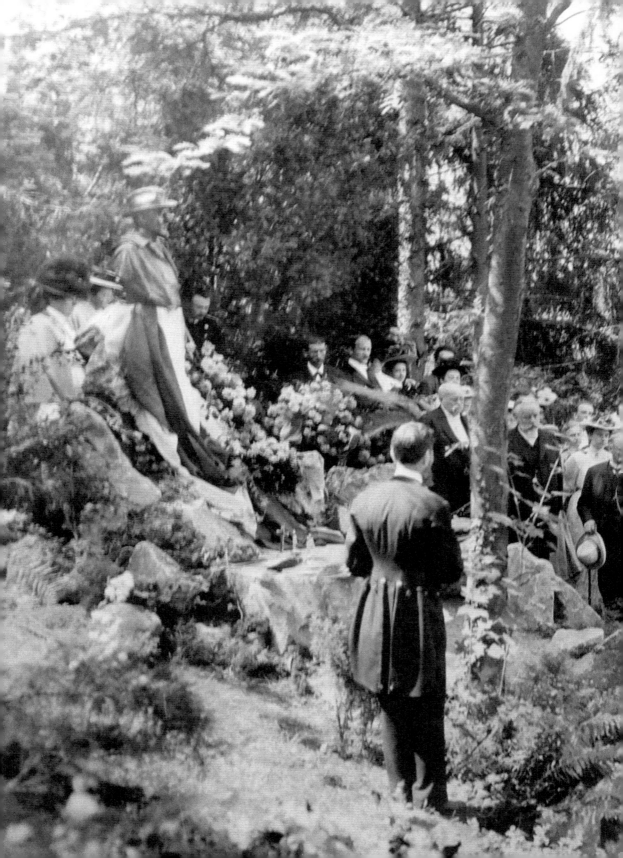

Anton Chekhov documented his final days at a sanatorium in Germany in 1904, and his account reflects the experience of many sanatorium patients at the time. The Russian writer and doctor had been plagued intermittently by tuberculosis for twenty years, but had avoided medical intervention. As he wrote to a friend early on, "The idea of having to undergo treatment and fuss over my physical condition produces in me something akin to revulsion. I'm not going to be treated." He also chose to keep his illness secret. In a sharp letter from 1897 he requested his brother's silence: "Nobody knows anything about my illness at home, so rein in your customary malice and don't blab about it in your letters." By some accounts even his wife, Olga, was unaware of his long battle with the disease until it returned, killing him at the age of 44.

Chekhov's Champagne

At the western edge of the Black Forest, Chekhov lay in bed at the Sommer Hotel in the spa town of Badenweiler and coughed into a spittoon that fitted into his pocket. He was skeptical of the institution's peculiar methods, but had reached the end of his resistance. In a letter he described daily life at the sanatorium with wry resignation:

"*Inside and outside not a sound to be heard; only at 7am and noon music plays in the park. The place is expensive but very talentless. I cannot fathom a drop of talent, not a drop of good taste in anything, but my orderliness and honesty are in excess... German doctors turned my life upside down: at 7am I take tea in bed—for some reason it has to be in bed; at 7.30 a sort of a German masseur comes and rubs me down with water and it turns out quite pleasant. Then I have to stay in bed for a while, then get up and at 8 I must drink acorn cocoa and eat an enormous quantity of butter. At 10, [I have] an extremely flavourful and aromatic puréed porridge, quite unlike ours. At 4pm, cocoa again, at 7 dinner. A cup of wild strawberry tisane is brought before bed—to induce sleep. All this has much of quackery in it, but also has much good and truly useful, e.g. porridge.*"

On the summer night that he died, his doctor sent for a bottle of champagne and a glass as a customary last rite. "He picked up the glass," Chekhov's wife recounted, "turned to me, smiled his wonderful smile and said, 'It's been such a long time since I've had champagne.'" He drained the full glass, sank back onto the bed, and was still.

continued from overleaf — **Ceremony held in memory of Anton Chehov, Badenweiler, Germany, circa 1908.**

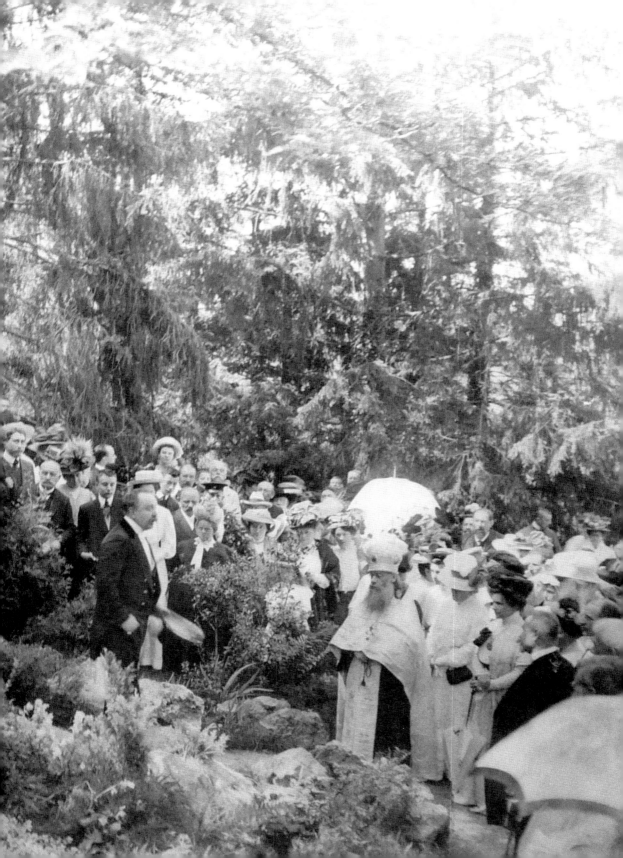

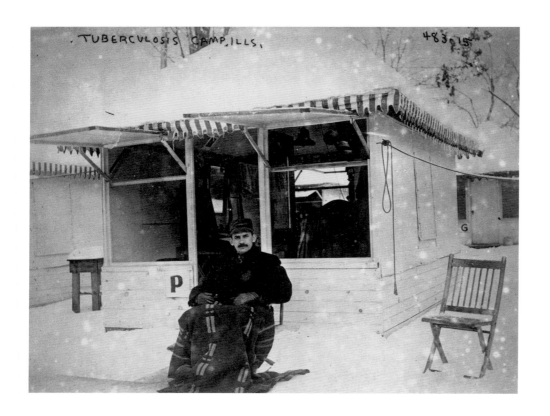

TUBERCULOSIS CAMP, ILLS.

483-15

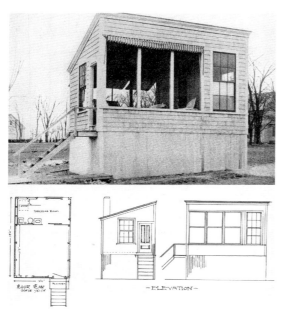

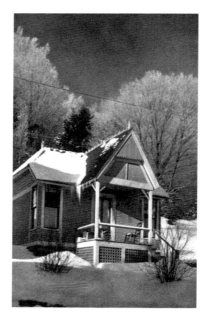

top — Man, with blanket over lap, seated in front of a small building in a tuberculosis camp. Ottawa, Illinois, circa 1908. bottom left — Tuberculosis hospital and sanatorium construction plan, circa 1911. bottom right — The Little Red Cottage, Adirondack Cottage Sanitarium (now Trudeau Sanatorium), Saranac Lake, New York.

COTTAGE CURES

Before the sanatorium cure made its way out west, it was first popularized in the United States in 1885, when Dr. Edward Livingston Trudeau opened his Adirondack Cottage Sanitarium in the thickly wooded mountains of northern New York state. A few years earlier, the young doctor, who had a lean build, a dark moustache surging into sideburns, and a grave diagnosis of pulmonary tuberculosis, said goodbye to his wife and children. He was going, as he later wrote, to "bury myself in the Adirondacks." Trudeau assumed his final months were upon him; any hope was crushed by the memory of helplessly witnessing the same disease kill his younger brother. He described the region he was entering as "an unbroken wilderness, and considered most dangerous for a chest invalid," but he loved the dazzling landscape dearly. He stayed at a lodge amid the white pines and pursued "an open-air life in the great forest." To his surprise, he survived and regained his health.

Trudeau read extensively about European sanatoriums and sought to institute a similar practice in the United States. The tranquil location on the shore of Saranac Lake, where he had lain for many days under the tall trees gazing out at the water, presented itself as ideal for treating patients. "I then unfolded... my plan of building a few cottages at Saranac Lake... where I could test Brehmer's and Dettweiler's rest, open-air, and sanatorium methods."[4] Trudeau's first patients were two ailing factor workers, the sisters Alice and Mary Hunt, who lived in a crowded New

4. Dr. Peter Dettweiler, one of Brehmer's patients healed by a six-year stay at Görbersdorf, left to found the Falkenstein sanatorium in 1876 in Germany's Taunus Mountains. Where Brehmer emphasized vigorous blood-pumping exercises for invalids, Dettweiler pioneered the rest cure—an approach that would prove more enduring. His sanatorium provided deep verandas and cane couches for patients to recline on while benefiting from the mountain air. He also founded Germany's first 'people's sanatorium' for invalids of low income—a model that would proliferate across the nation and beyond.

York City tenement. Their passage and treatment was paid for by charitable donations, and they arrived "in wretched health, poorly clad to stand the Adirondack winter cold, and nearly dead with fatigue." The sisters were housed in a one-room wooden cottage nicknamed 'Little Red' (which still exists), and encouraged to eat well, rest, and take in gallons of fresh air on the small porch. Their health improved greatly. Although they eventually died from tuberculosis, Trudeau was certain that their lives were lengthened by his treatment.

From these humble beginnings Trudeau purchased 90 acres on the lake with the help of investors. His institution grew, with buildings for administration, research, caregiver training, and a laboratory with the latest medical equipment. Wanting to avoid a massive building with dark hallways and small windows, like Brehmer's Gothic building in Görbersdorf, Trudeau chose the homier style of 'cure cottages.' These houses varied in style and size, from a gingerbread Queen Anne look to Swiss chalet to English countryside, but all required the crucial features of effective air circulation and outdoor space for reposing. Some cure cottages were newly built, while other, already existing houses were updated to include screen doors and broad decks.

The rules of Trudeau's institution were strict: alcohol, smoking, cursing, and intimate relations were forbidden. (The phrase 'cousining' referred to illicit romantic affairs among patients; a secluded gazebo on the grounds was called the "cousinola.") The doldrums of open-air reclining were alleviated with mandatory arts and crafts classes, formal dinners, and an enforced culture of optimism. To strengthen this sense of community, the sanatorium launched a magazine, the *Journal of The Outdoor Life*, in 1904. Informative and briskly encouraging, it included reports on medical discoveries, patient testimonials, and a cornucopia of advertisements for the long-term invalid, from a laundry service that specialized in disinfecting to nutritious malted milk to 'window tents'—devices that enabled a patient to put their head out of a window while keeping warm below the neck. Trudeau's patients didn't use window tents as they were able to recline outdoors, even during the icy winter, swaddled in blankets and fur. They lay in the newly invented Adirondack cure chair (not to be confused with the famed Adirondack deck chair): a padded chaise longue based on a German sanatorium model, equipped with wheels and a swiveling desk surface for books or letter writing.

Trudeau's sanatorium grew in reputation, despite the uneven success of his methods. He only accepted patients in the very earliest stages of the disease, some of whom would have improved anyway. Many curious doctors and health officials visited his Adirondack Cottage Sanatorium, and soon the doctor's methods were replicated across the country. Word was also spread by patients with some celebrity. The author Robert Louis Stevenson, for example, found his health greatly improved at Saranac Lake and often recommended this "American Davos."

However, not every 'lunger' (as some tuberculars called themselves) could afford to travel to sanatoriums and pay the fees for room, board, and medical treatment. A network of free sanatoriums paid for by charitable, religious or government institutions emerged, but beds filled quickly. Instead, the majority of the afflicted were cared for at home by relatives, despite the looming threat of contagion. Or, if they could afford the train ticket and survive the journey, they might relocate to the natural sanatorium of America's Southwest.

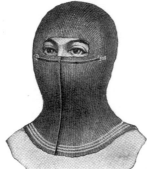

VISOR HOOD AND MUFFLER

Patented in Canada March 22, 1904   Pat. in United States Aug. 30, 1904

This splendid invention will be found a veritable godsend to all those who spend considerable time in the open air during the winter months. Whether for use during the day or night it will be found the most perfect protection against the cold for the head, face and neck ever devised.

Please Note the Following Points of Excellence:

1. Simply as a neck muffler and chest protector, it is the best of its kind on the market.
2. The muffler can instantly be converted into a hood and face protector.
3. The hood, being elastic throughout, fits any head like a glove.
4. Two hooks and a strong elastic adjust the face opening to any size.
5. The eyes, ears, mouth and nose have absolute freedom, even when the face is completely covered.
6. It is impossible to feel cold in it even in the severest weather.
7. The breath goes through the material. It does not interfere with free respiration.
8. As a driving or sleeping cap it is worth its weight in gold.
9. We knit it from the best, pure-wool yarns, imported directly from England.
10. Made in black and navy only. **Sent postpaid, to any address upon receipt of $1.50.** State color preferred.

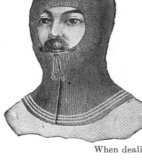

Address

VISOR KNITTING CO.,
Niagara Falls,
New York

When dealing with Advertisers please mention Journal of The Outdoor Life.

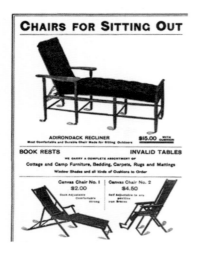

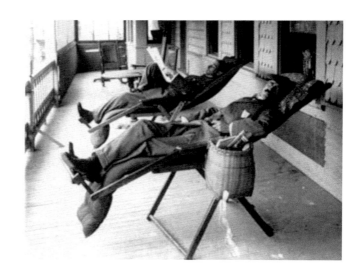

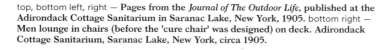

top, bottom left, right — Pages from the *Journal of The Outdoor Life,* published at the Adirondack Cottage Sanitarium in Saranac Lake, New York, 1905. bottom right — Men lounge in chairs (before the 'cure chair' was designed) on deck. Adirondack Cottage Sanitarium, Saranac Lake, New York, circa 1905.

'The Walker Portable Cottage

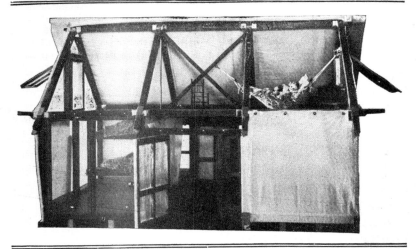

ABSOLUTELY MOSQUITO PROOF   **STORM CURTAINS AND WIRE SCREENS FOR ALL OPENINGS**

An Ideal Outing Cottage, Can be Set Up Ready for Occupancy in Two Hours

A Home for Six People $100.00

This does not include attic floor or beds. See price list

This frame is covered with 10 oz. Army Duck.   Three pieces cover this building. This is not a tent, but a substantial frame that can be sided up and shingled, if desired.   Each piece drops into place, and the two rods shown in cut locks the frame.   No bolts, screws or nails to remove.   This cut represents a cottage 12x18 feet and will furnish sleeping room for 16 people, giving each one a good spring bed 2½x6 feet. Nine dressing rooms 6x6 feet each. Thoroughly ventilated.

JAS. A. WALKER, Inventor and Manufacturer, 215 N. Court St., **Rockford, Ill.**

When dealing with Advertisers please mention Journal of The Oudoor Life.

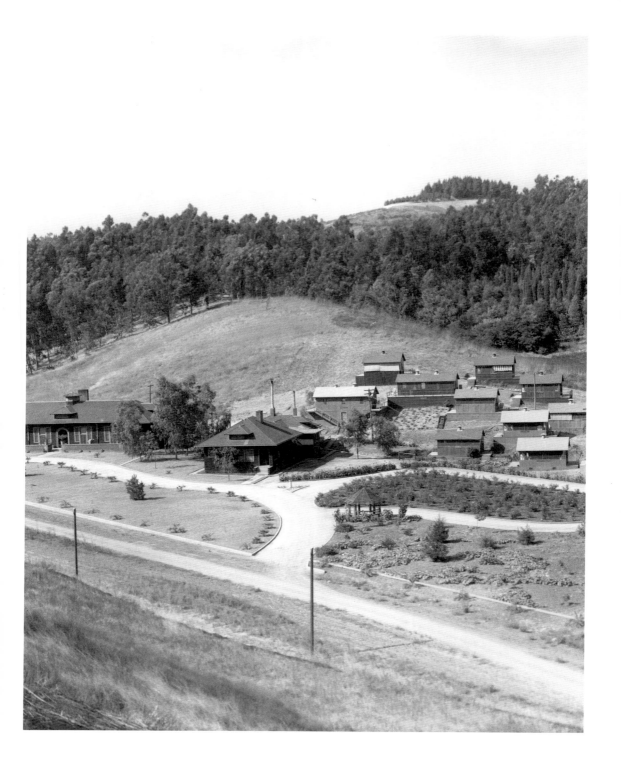

above — **Panoramic view of the Barlow Sanatorium in Elysian Park, Los Angeles, California, circa 1915.**

In 1880, much of Southern California outside of Downtown Los Angeles was still a quiet landscape of sleepy ranches dotted with adobe homes and dusty unpaved roads. But the decade saw enormous change as newcomers poured into the city, increasing the population seven times over.

New homes, roads, schools, churches and hotels were rapidly built, and irrigation systems greened the parched ground into a verdant patchwork of orchards and farmland. Countless health-hotels, boarding houses, lunger colonies, and varieties of nature-cures also spread across the land, forming what became known as the 'Sanatorium Belt'.

One of the early boarding houses that took in consumptives was opened in 1882 by Emma C. Bangs, who came to Pasadena to help her ill daughter. Bangs had a two-story wooden house built overlooking a deep dry gulch. She then began taking in tenants, many of whom came for the winter season. One resident, a Mrs. Jennie Banbury Ford, recounted this remarkable anecdote:

"When Mrs. Bangs' boarding house was most flourishing, there were many consumptives coming and going. It became so depressing it was suggested that they band themselves together under the head of "the busted lung brigade," and create more hopeful and cheerful feeling. The suggestion was carried out and proved very successful. They elected officers, had a beautiful silk banner with "B.L.B." embroidered on it and met all "busted lungers" with open arms. Those whose stay was ended were started on their several ways with smiles and cheers. Each member was compelled to sign the by-laws, which were amusing at least. They must not sit in a draft, must consume just so much milk and so many eggs each day and look after each other's comfort, etc. To help the fun along, Mrs. Bangs bought a parrot in

Los Angeles who knew how to cough exactly like a "lunger" and con-
tributed much to the amusement. I don't believe a more grotesque club
ever existed, do you? It lasted for several years."

The cheerfulness of the B.L.B. aside, most health seekers
had a less jubilant time. The high population of invalids had
attracted a flood of doctors, or those posing as such, whose
methods of healing were often eccentric and unregulated.
Attempts to establish a state medical board faced fierce and
constant resistance. Its first (of several) iterations, in the
late 1870s, included three separate licenses: for conventional
medicine, eclectic medicine[5], and homeopathic medicine.
Unfortunately, it was impossible to pursue and fine the scores of
unlicensed practitioners, some of whom vocally objected to the
very notion of being tested and licensed in the first place. "In
a country where sickness was once almost unknown," observed
British novelist Horace A. Vachell, "doctors, dentists, faith-
healers, and quacks multiply and increase as the quails of
yore." If one went without a doctor's care, by choice or lack of
finances, it was often up to the invalid and their caretaker to
perambulate from inland heat to coastal mist, mountain pines
to valley shade, bravely experimenting with atmospheres like
ingredients to be measured and decanted into an airy elixir.

Charles D. Willard was a thin, serious-looking young writer
whose battle with consumption brought him, reluctantly, to Los
Angeles in 1888. As he strained toward stable health he wrote
hundreds of letters home from boarding houses in this "hope-
lessly vulgar" city to his family in Chicago, whom he missed
inconsolably. He found work in publishing and at the newly
revived Los Angeles Chamber of Commerce, where his literary
aspirations led him to co-found *The Land of Sunshine,* a promotional magazine extolling the region's riches.

In 1891 the return of his wracking cough led him and his
wife Mary to move to a more rural area. He described their new
domicile in Glendale as "a small village eight miles west of town
up among the mountains" which would "be vastly better for our
healths." Willard tried to maintain a sanguine tone, describing
"lots of flowers and shrubbery" around their house and his

hopes that the new location would enable him "to get some out-of-door life" and "get toned up." He also resurrected his habit of bathing in ice-cold water each morning, a routine that sometimes helped immensely, and at other times made him worse.

A few years later the Willards' baby daughter Florence took ill, and they ventured to the coast some 22 miles away. He wrote: "We tried Santa Monica for a few days and it helped her so that we go down on the first of the month." Florence improved, and as she grew up was taught the healthy habits of sleeping outdoors and practicing gymnastics regularly. Despite his discreet battle with illness, Willard worked his way into the city's influential circles. He was a notably dapper man, although his attention to dress might have been a means to distract from his forebodingly weak physique. He poured what strength he had into producing reams of inflated rhetoric about the salubrity of Southern California while suffering greatly, often writing from his sick bed, never recovering full health.

As the nineteenth century drew to a close, news of tuberculosis's airborne nature was disseminated widely through public health campaigns, amplifying its danger. Historian Emily K. Abel points out in *Suffering in the Land of Sunshine: A Los Angeles Illness Narrative*, that by "spreading the message that contact with a tubercular could be deadly, health educators transformed sufferers into menaces." Panic spread faster than the deadly bacilli. Willard had no trouble finding lodging at boarding houses or hotels, or renting houses during the 1880s and '90s, even with a constant hacking cough and face gaunt with illness. But after a fire destroyed his house in 1910, this family man with influential friends discovered that "everybody

5. Homeopathic medicine involves taking small daily doses of a natural substance that would induce similar symptoms to the disease. "Eclectic" medicine, a term in use from about 1830 to 1930, referred to a theory of botanical treatments and physical therapy, but was also used to encompass anything that wasn't conventional.

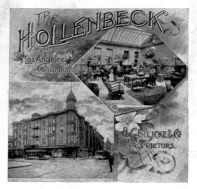
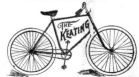

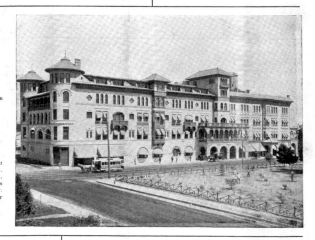
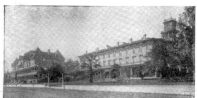

readers may be getting acquainted with it. In its new form this will be far ,and away the handsomest periodical ever issued in Southern California, as it intends to be the most readable. In artistic and literary quality it will be something we shall not have to smuggle out of sight when we hear the footsteps of an Easterner. It will also give him more varied and more valuable information about this country than any monthly publication has ever given. And it will not make him think he would better fetch along a schoolmaster when he comes to visit us.

The new cover will speak for itself as well to the artistic as to the general eye. Simple and strong, original but not eccentric, significant and appropriate yet highly decorative, it proves itself no journeyman job. Most magazines are limited, by the very breadth of their field, to the purely conventional symbols. The most expressive hallmark they can find to typify their locale, their character, their scope, is a rococo tidy, a pair of Corinthian gateposts, or a Wenzell young lady who changes her dress once a month.

But our more definite if narrower field is more generous of artistic suggestions. The peculiar fitness of the California lion — the most perfect of the animate creation in the New World, the highest type of physical grace and sinewy strength, the most typical sun-lover — as the fetich of Southern California was outlined in the April number. He is a symbol worth having, as Mr. Borglum has drawn him basking Sphinx-like in the setting sun.

The rose is as perfectly typical, not only of fertility but of refinement. As the king of beasts stands for physical, so does the queen of flowers for mental, grace. There are no roses where man is uncultivated; and while California is not the only country where roses grow, it is the one where they reach their highest perfection.

The legend — that apt old Spanish proverb: "the lands of the sun expand the soul" — was kindly suggested for the magazine by W. C. Brownell, the well-known New York critic and literary adviser to the Scribners.

John Gutzon Borglum, who has interpreted the design with so firm a hand, adds another little touch to its aptness. The editor of this magazine was among the first to see and predict a large future for the crude boy who ten years ago was making in this city his first art beginnings, with all things against him except one. Since then, by no adventitious circumstance but by sheer talent, he has conquered honor not only in his own country but in several others; and today it is not an unknown lad but an associate of the Salon Champ de Mars, Paris, who draws the cover of the LAND OF SUNSHINE.

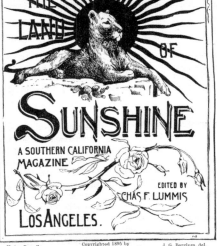

Union Eng. Co.   Copyrighted 1895 by   J. G. Borglum, del.
              Land of Sunshine Publishing Co.
SKETCH OF THE NEW COVER FOR JUNE.

There is no such thing as "South California." There is a State of California; the more genial and more prosperous end of which is known as Southern California — just as the region of Fall River would be spoken of as Southern Massachusetts. "South California" would mean, to those who know the English language from a premature persimmon, that there were two States of California, as of Carolina.

There are not; and there never will be. We Californians glory in our State, whichever end we inhabit. Now and then there is skin-deep talk of splitting it; but that has no backing of public opinion. Nobody had ever thought of such a thing, but for the fact that this end of the State had always been despitefully entreated by the northern end. It is not pleasant to be unable to get justice. But the West as a whole is not going to secede from the Union because it is thus far impossible to beat into the skull of Washington a geography more than 500 miles wide. People who think, need hardly be reminded that until we outvote Northern California we cannot get ourselves amputated; that when we outvote them, we can make our own justice and shall no longer have the shadow of a wish to part with that enormous and superb area which is the proper complement to ours. The old name, California, means something; it suggests a story that every one knows. We cannot afford to part with it and its associations.

❋ ❋

This side of Bret Harte, no book of California stories ranks with Margaret Collier Graham's *Stories of the Foothills*, recently issued by Houghton, Mifflin & Co. More romantic "local color" has been put forth from this romantic State; but in literary art and human interest Mrs. Graham so easily distances the field that comparison would be uncomfortable; and in calm truth, she has as little to be ashamed in the best Eastern company as among California writers. The average of them that "rabbit the literary warren" reckon it quite superfluous to know whereof they write, and still wonder why the rivers refuse to kindle for them. In reading Mrs. Graham, one is as conscious of her grasp of the subject as of her self-control with it, and as of her swift, sinewy, clean-cut style, which would successfully carry a much inferior art. But while Mrs. Graham knows how to say it, she still more has something to say. The object of a story is not so much to pass muster with the critic as to interest the reader; and the reader who is not carried along by "The Withrow Water-Right" is not healthfully portable, that is all. Mrs. Graham is a long-time resident of Pasadena, western in the best and fullest sense, and as interesting as her stories.

slams the door in the face of the consumptive now." He died four years later at the age of 48, taking minor solace in the belief that his lifespan had been extended by the climate.

After years of advertising the region quite explicitly to lure invalids, residents now complained that promoting health services would only burden the area's resources. In 1902 the Los Angeles city council passed a law prohibiting hospitals from caring for consumptives within the city limits. The small nearby town of Sierra Madre, once the region's jewel of high-altitude and dry air in the foothills, passed an ordinance to limit tent houses and other healing institutions to "dispel the illusion... that this city is nothing but a big consumptive camp."

Tales circulated of penniless consumptives with multiple children in tow arriving by train and collapsing at the station. Charitable institutions and the free county hospital were overcapacity and understaffed. Eventually, locals lobbied for a law decreeing that only residents of at least one year could get free medical treatment, trying to ward off the steady flow of ill and impoverished newcomers. Suspicion and hostility were heaped upon non-white Californians especially, including native, Chinese, and Mexican laborers, who were viewed as likely carriers of the disease. "We wish more population of the right sort," read a coded editorial in *The Land of Sunshine*, "But we are particular. We are anxious to have our friends come; but not everybody."

In order to contain the disease, consumptives were encouraged to enter sanatoriums skirting the city, staffed with doctors and nurses enforcing their unique diets and strict daily schedules. One of the first was Barlow Sanatorium, founded in 1902 by New York doctor Dr. Walter Jarvis Barlow, who had come west to aid his own case of tuberculosis. Barlow married an heiress to a locomotive fortune and they hosted parties to raise funds for a small, low-cost sanatorium for "indigent consumptives." The patients were housed in secluded bungalows in the hills of the Echo Park neighborhood. They started each day with a plunge into cold water, were forbidden to spit, and lights were turned out at nine o'clock. Each evening the patients' handkerchiefs were burned. Once Barlow's patients were strong enough, they were made to work the grounds, to improve both their health and their ability to contribute to society after release. And although the doctor started with just two patients, his sanatorium grew to accommodate over 40 and acquired a long waiting list.

A year later, the higher-cost Pottenger Sanatorium, set amid fragrant citrus groves on a southern mountain slope, opened with eleven beds. Its founder, Dr. Francis M. Pottenger, had traveled to Southern California with his wife in an attempt to cure her consumption. As his wife's health failed, Pottenger devoted himself to researching the disease and its possible cures. Influenced by reading about the success of Brehmer's and Trudeau's methods and traveling to observe their institutions in Görbersdorf and Saranac Lake, he decided to build his own sanatorium, suited to the unique, health-giving climate at home.

"My task," recalled Pottenger, "was to adapt the buildings to the year-round open-air life in Southern California." To this end he housed patients in canvas tents open on three sides, walled in by wire netting. No thick walls, elaborate ventilation systems or fur blankets were required. The doctor also had unorthodox plans for the interior. "When I gave the architect my ideas about the central building, with rooms only on one side of the hall and large bay windows in each room, he said, 'It will look like hell and the cost per room will be almost doubled.'" But Pottenger prevailed, and the resulting exposure to sunlight and air, as well as a diet of garden-grown vegetables, fresh dairy, and copious doses of the 'Pottenger cocktail' (orange juice, soda, and castor oil) proved beneficial. Due to its modern methods and strong recovery rate, his institution gained widespread prestige and influence. By 1911 there were at least twenty-three sanatoriums throughout California, and a few years later those that accepted lower-income patients began receiving state funds.

Nonetheless, the reputation of Southern California's miracle climate was being steadily eclipsed by a drive to redefine the region's identity. Working in tandem with a slew of laws tracking or excluding consumptives, promotional publications shifted gears. Now they hawked the miracles of plentiful business opportunities and cheap land, hoping to lure hearty, industrious families instead of the weak and dying. Southern California was recast as a place where the healthy could get even healthier. If an orange grew into a remarkably vibrant globe in the dead of winter, if the oldest and largest trees in the nation soared from Californian soil, what then might happen to a person of good health?

No longer were desperate invalids free to investigate curative microclimates or fill brocaded hotel hallways with the pathos of their coughs. The region was growing up; its years of unregulated health-seeking were drawing to a close.

top — Pottenger Sanatorium, Monrovia, California, circa 1923.
bottom — Dr. F. M. Pottenger, Sr. at his sanatorium, circa 1903.

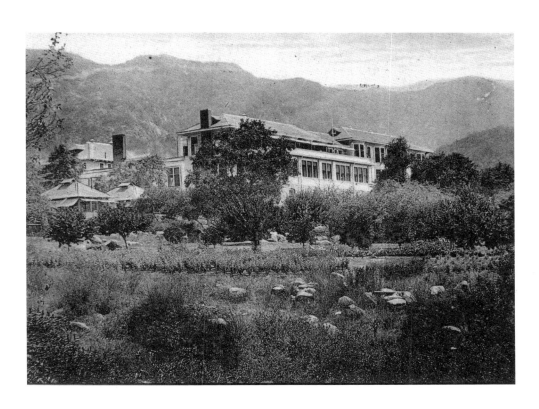

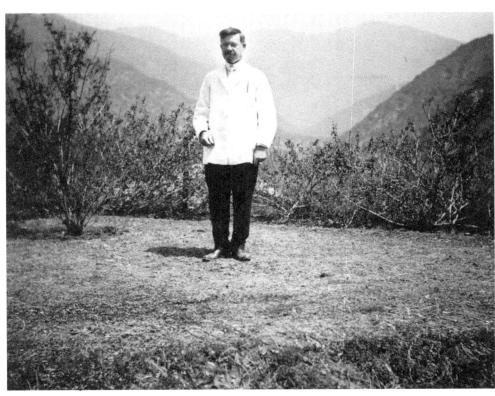

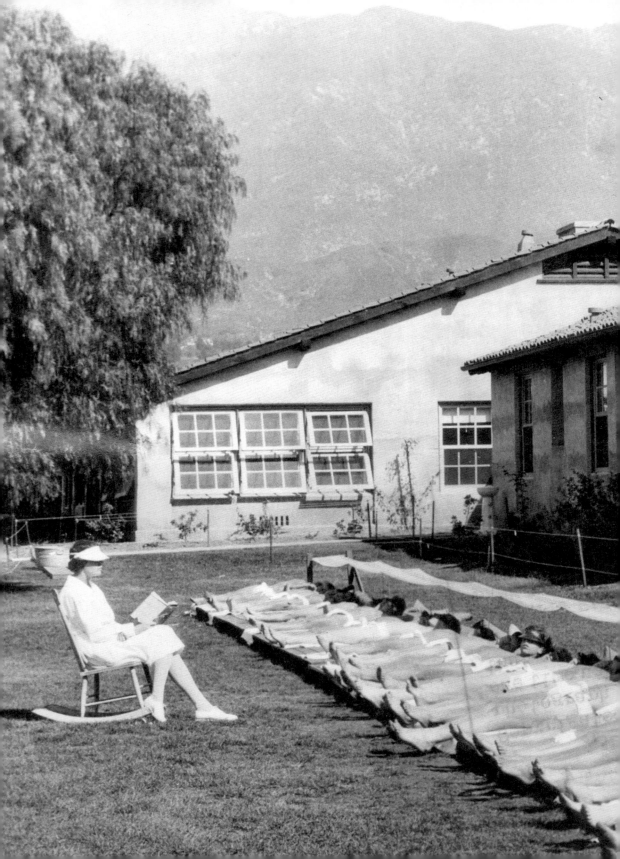

T he Roman writer Pliny is said to have stated, "the sun is the best remedy." Ancient Arabic and Roman doctors prescribed exposure to the sun for a wide range of ailments. But for centuries, upper-class Europeans avoided the sun, seeking to keep their skin as pale as possible to distinguish it from the bronzed look of laborers. That changed with the resurgence of nature cures, in particular sun cures. In 1889 Dr. J. Orgeas of Cannes, France, wrote:

"Just as the Sun is the principle of all life, so it is the source of all healing. It is the Sun, and uniquely the Sun, that sick people seek in winter on our coast. It is the Great Doctor, Doctor of the Faculty of the Sky, to whom the suffering come to demand a cure for their ills."

Late nineteenth-century doctors promoted the ancient, quasi-mystical origins of light therapy while simultaneously advocating for it as a modern scientific method. The eccentric Swiss naturopath Arnold Rikli—whose credo was "Water is good, air is better, and light is best of all"—is credited with introducing medicinal sunbathing at his two clinics in Slovenia and Italy in the 1850s. Physicians knew that the sun could kill bacteria; it followed that it could kill disease. Sun exposure was later given medical credence by the Danish scientist Niels Ryberg Finsen, who won the 1903 Nobel Prize in physiology for his research into the healing effects phototherapy had on ailments such as lupus vulgaris.

Influenced by Finsen, several doctors brought helio- and phototherapies to their clinics, often employing them in peculiar ways. American doctor and Christian health evangelist Dr. John Harvey Kellogg visited Finsen at his Light Institute in Copenhagen twice, and employed light therapies at his sanatorium in Battle Creek, Michigan. Kellogg's patients were rolled into his Horizontal Incandescent Light Cabinet (an ornate wooden contraption that acted like a tanning bed). Others lay under a massive metal octopus-like machine, whose telescoping legs emitted focused doses of "electrophototherapy." Kellogg himself often wore an all-white suit, believing it enabled him to absorb more sunlight—especially the ultraviolet rays he considered most salubrious.

In Switzerland, Dr. Auguste Rollier supervised famous heliocentric clinics in the village of Leysin, near Lake Geneva. There, adults and children were sent out into the mountains in all seasons, clad only in white loincloths and sheets. Those who were confined to a bed were wheeled out onto broad porches to drink the dazzling alpine rays. The author of influential manifestos on heliotherapy, Rollier was called "The High Priest of Modern Sun-Worshippers."

As more doctors and institutions embraced sun cures, the variety of treatments grew. Some clinics, following Rollier's methods, carefully exposed patients' bodies inch-by-inch to the light for a carefully measured number of minutes per day. A clinic in the South of France prescribed nude lolling on outdoor mattresses, with regular turnings of the body.

While light therapy was essentially jettisoned with the introduction of modern antibiotics in the 1940s, recent medical research has proved that the fervor for sunlight may have been on the right track. The impact of vitamin D on healthy bones has been known for decades. (Before the Second World War a synthetic form of vitamin D was added to milk, greatly reducing cases of rickets, which had plagued residents of the northern cities of Europe and North America.) But in the 1980s it was discovered that vitamin D was beneficial to all of the internal organs, helping to prevent certain cancers, fight infections, and regulate diabetes. There are now dozens of recent scientific studies that prove vitamin D was indeed able to fight, if not eliminate, tubercle bacilli. Scientists have also concluded that vitamin D is produced when the skin is exposed to ultraviolet B (UVB) light, and this is best absorbed when the sun is high in the sky. In northern regions of higher latitudes, the decrease in the sun's height means that even if one was to sunbathe all winter long, the body would not absorb enough UVB. So southern migrants and sun-cure advocates were right. It just took a century for science to prove it.

continued from overleaf — **Boys sunbathing circa 1928 at an open-air "preventorium," a school for "pre-tubercular" boys that opened in 1922 in Pasadena.**

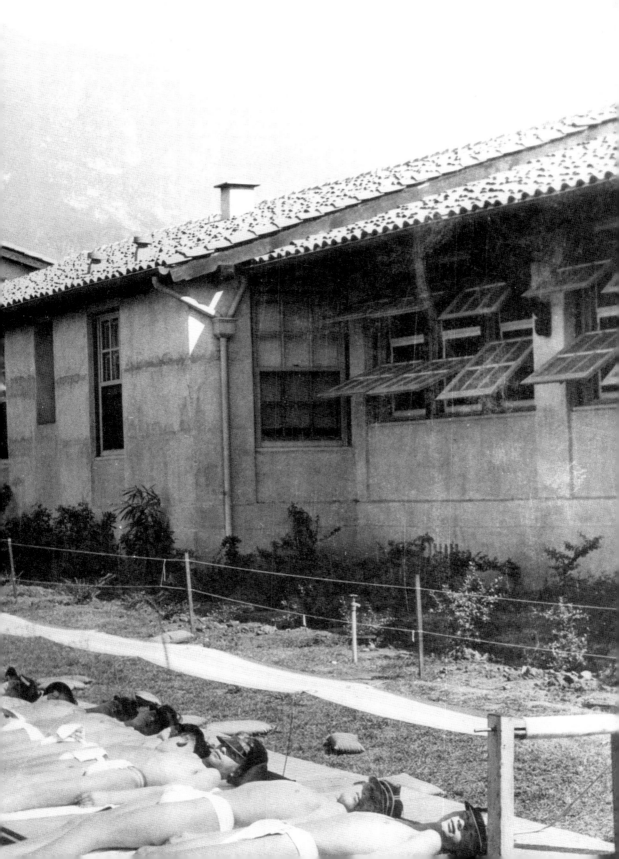

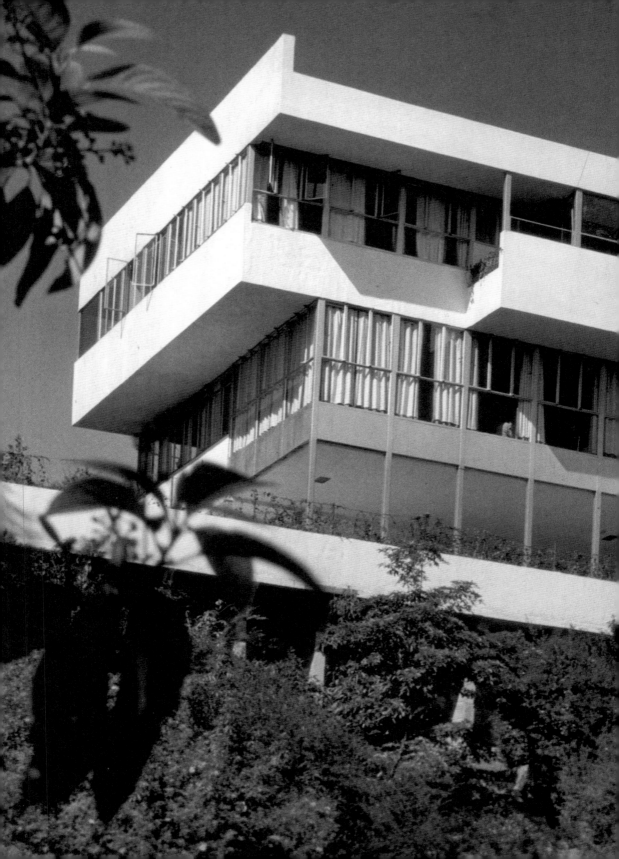

Building a Cure

"The machine that we live in is an old coach full of tuberculosis... whereas the [modern] house is a [health] machine for living."

Le Corbusier, vis-à-vis Margaret Campbell

previous page — **View of the Lovell 'Health House' designed by Richard Neutra.**

Imagine a 'modern house' for a moment. One usually summons white walls. Sharp angles. Wide spans of glass. Minimalist decor. Some people dislike the aesthetic because it feels cold or clinical. Indeed, at least in its beginnings, the modern house was meant to feel clinical, a clean structure opening toward light, sun, and health. Or a "machine for living," as Swiss architect Le Corbusier famously declared in 1923. Decades later, historian and designer Margaret Campbell added to his statement: a house was a machine for living, yes, while a modern house was a health machine.

For years the city, the slum, and the overstuffed, dimly lit house had been blamed for breeding disease and degrading wellbeing. The common solution, for those who were able, was to flee, seeking recuperation in a medical institution or healthier clime. But eventually the perceived source of the problem—the design of buildings—came under scrutiny. Following the lead of sanatoriums, buildings began to be reevaluated in light of new beliefs about hygiene and healing.

In an unusual partnership doctors, city planners, public health officials, and architects were allied in their pursuit of building reform. This was evident at all scales by the 1920s, from mass housing for the working classes to factories, schools, and private homes built for wealthy, health-focused patrons. Such attempts to position design *as a cure* also resulted in some unusual experimental ideas, as we will see.

"Modern architecture can be argued to have been shaped by the dominant medical obsession of its time: tuberculosis," writes architectural historian Beatriz Colomina. "It is as though the widespread success of modern architecture depended on its association with health, its internationalism the consequence of the global spread of the disease it was meant to resist." She's referring in part to the International Style, a type of architectural Modernism that gelled in the 1920s and '30s and has dominated our notion

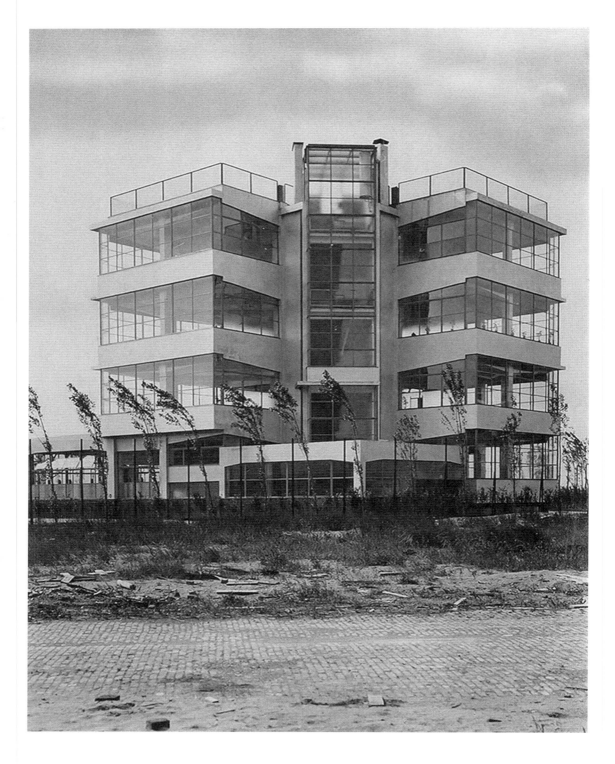

above — **Duiker's Open Air School, Amsterdam, the Netherlands.** top right — **Dr. Saidman's Solarium Tournant (turning solarium), Aix-les-Bains, France.** bottom right — **Zonnestraal Sanatorium, Hilversum, the Netherlands.**

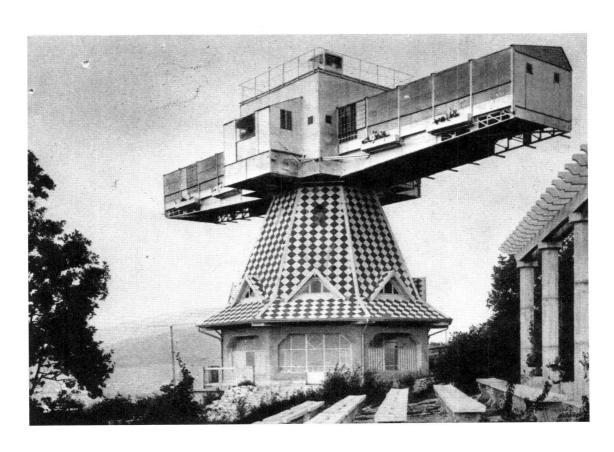

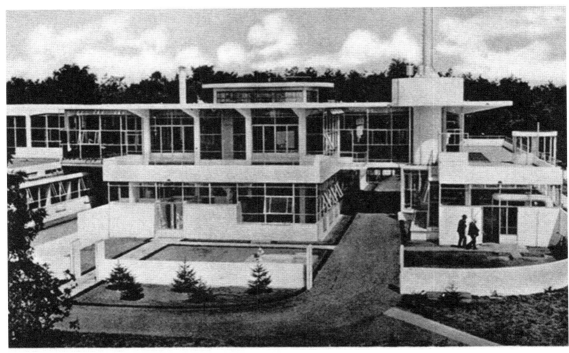

of 'modern' to this day. Usually constructed of glass and steel, the style was defined by rectilinear forms, unadorned surfaces, open interiors, and a weightless quality. In short, it defined the now-familiar trope of a sparse, clean design whose current ubiquity—seen in the pages of magazines like *Dwell* and *Wallpaper**, or in cold corporate boardrooms—belies its original ability to shock.

In subsequent decades the modern house became a marker of luxury and status, but Colomina notes that at the time of its emergence, "the fear of illness was more important for people than the alleged beauty of a modern white wall." The white wall had an important purpose: to reveal dirt, or rather, to display an absence of dirt—a sanitized surface clean as alpine snow. Glass walls and balconies invited exposure to healing sunlight. An open-plan interior enabled air circulation. The rationality and deliberateness would be as effective as a machine—the *echt* modern object.

These design elements had long been gestating in sanatorium architecture. Lavish hotels added balconies and terraces while cottages were reconceived with walls of screens or canvas flaps. The design of sanatoriums kept pace with changing ideas of healthfulness: more nature, more air, more sunlight. (Recall Thomas Mann's description in *The Magic Mountain* of the many-balconied Swiss sanatorium, so porous as to resemble a sponge.)

Influential design books from the late 1920s focused on the vital need for sunlight and air, and their surveys of new architecture seamlessly moved between sanatoriums, houses, and gymnasiums.[1] It could be hard to tell one from the other. As Colomina asserts, "Modern architecture was literally presented and understood as a piece of medical equipment." Her statement at first evokes something cold and metallic. But medical equipment, at the time, could mean any tool that caught sunlight.

Le Corbusier, an ardent sunbather, was fixated on hygienic, solar-centric design. He proclaimed that a house should be considered a "daughter of the sun," and his designs were profoundly attuned to the reception of sunlight. "Doling out cosmic energy," he stated, "the sun's effects are both physical and moral, and they have been too much neglected in recent times. The results of that neglect can be seen in cemetery and sanatorium." A true heliophile, Le Corbusier wrote poems celebrating sunlight and made drawings and paintings exalting the sun's arc in relation to buildings. ('Father of heliotherapy' Dr. Auguste Rollier claimed that Le Corbusier was influenced by seeing his heliotherapy clinics in Leysin.)

The hygienic focus of sanatoriums influenced the architecture of many building types, including the domestic 'daughters of the sun.' It also resulted in at least two remarkable offshoots: one, a brief and eccentric foray into heliotropic design, the other, an elegant stride forward in the course of Modernist architecture.

First, the curious case of the heliotropic building. By 1905 several small one-room rotating sheds had been built on the grounds of sanatoriums in Switzerland, England, and Scotland. In Davos they were called 'sunboxes.' Fully opened to the elements on one side, the sheds could be moved along a metal track to follow the arc of the sun. Easy to purchase and assemble, revolving sheds for domestic use were sold by greenhouse and garden hut companies.[2] One English company claimed that their revolving huts "enabled

---

1. See, for example, critic Sigfried Giedion's *Befreites Wohnen* (*Freed Living*), the cover of which is a photograph of a glass wall and terrace beyond, with the German words for 'light', 'air', and 'opening' overlaid repeatedly. Or architect Richard Döcker's*Terrasentyp: Krankenhaus, Erholungsheim, Hotel, Bürohaus, Einfamiliënhaus Siedlungshaus, Miethaus und die Stadt* (*Types of Terraces:* *Hospital, rest home, hotel, office building, one-family house housing estate, rental house and the city*) in which he proclaims, "The old traditional form of the closed and finished building block has been exploded, the world enclosed inside the house bursts out and forces its way toward the light and sun, seeking to merge with nature and the landscape."

2. English playwright and polemicist George Bernard Shaw used a small three-walled rotating garden hut mounted on a turntable at his home in Hertfordshire as a writing studio for decades. In a 1929 article, the hut was called an "aid to health," describing how Shaw nudged it around with his shoulder until the sun streamed inside.

BUILDING A CURE

the most delicate to take the utmost advantage of fresh air and sunshine, whilst strong and cold winds are excluded."

By the 1930s the logic of the heliotropic structure resulted in the construction of the bizarre Solarium Tournant, an open-air hospital mounted on the top of an octagonal windmill base in Aix-les-Bains, France. A good example of an architect-doctor partnership was when Romanian-French specialist in X-ray and UV light therapies, Dr. Jean Saidman, collaborated with architect André Farde. Together they built two rotating clinics in France and one for an intrigued maharaja in Gujarat, India (which still stands). Patients received various types of concentrated natural and artificial light treatments as their room slowly traced a wide circle in the sky, following the sun.

At the other end of the spectrum were sanatoriums raised to stunning aesthetic heights. They may not have rotated on metal gears, but they nonetheless operated as highly functional machines. The two most celebrated examples are the Zonnestraal Sanatorium in Hilversum, the Netherlands, and Paimio Sanatorium near Turku, in Southwest Finland, both constructed during the late 1920s-early 30s. They are today counted among the most significant modern buildings of the twentieth century.

Zonnestraal, which means 'sunbeam' in Dutch, was designed by Johannes Duiker and Bernard Bijvoet for diamond industry laborers suffering from tuberculosis and other respiratory ailments. White, lean, and nearly translucent, the sanatorium appears to be made almost entirely of glass, disappearing into its natural surroundings of heath and pine forest. Inside, the surfaces are painted pale blue, light yellow, and cream, bringing the buoyant colors of clear skies indoors. The buildings functioned with great efficiency, with every inch accounted for. A historian wrote that Zonnestraal's "dazzling white walls, huge shimmering

Playwright George Bernard Shaw in front of his rotating writer's hut, which he calls "The Shelter." St. Albans, Hertfordshire, England, circa 1946.

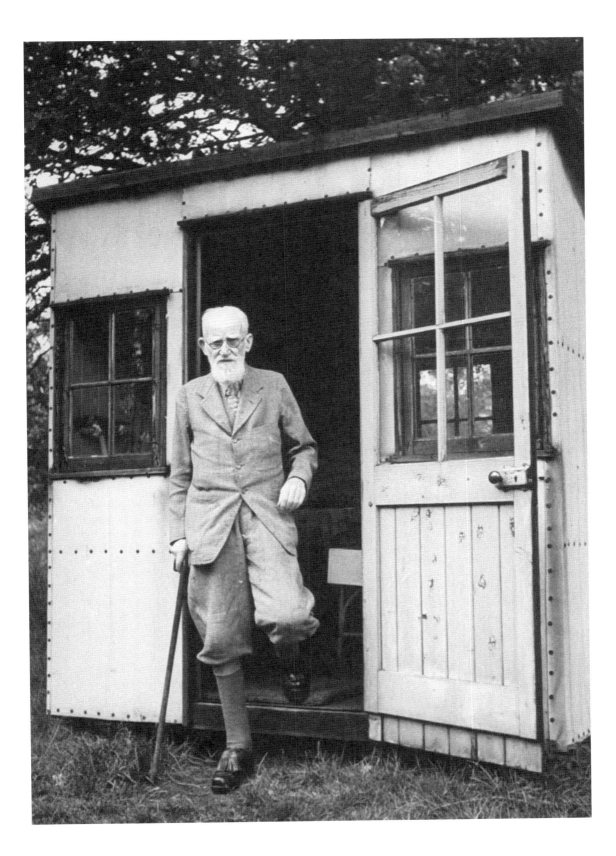

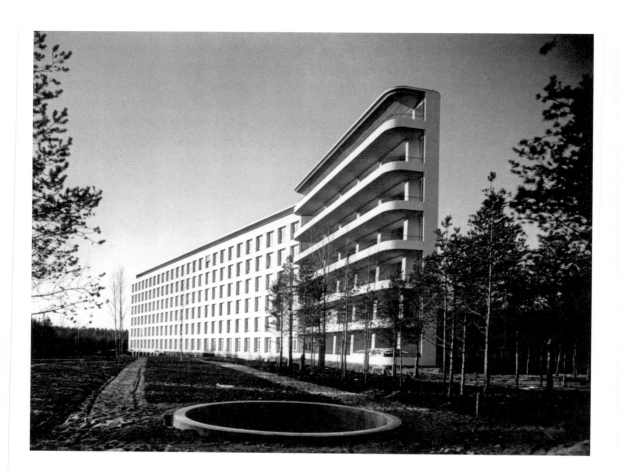

66   Paimio Sanatorium, Finland.

sheets of glass, and daring thin reinforced-concrete frame... evoked the construction of modern factories, ships, and aeroplanes—those paradigms of the 'clean machine' so often invoked in Modernist promotional texts." It was known locally as 'the white ship on the heath.'

One important visitor to Zonnestraal was Finnish architect Alvar Aalto, who also toured Duiker's Open-Air School for Healthy Children in Amsterdam, an impossibly airy stack of glass and spacious balconies completed in 1930. Duiker's buildings greatly impacted Aalto's design for Paimio Sanatorium. Rising over the canopy of the dense forest, wrapped in ribbons of white and glass, Aalto's seven-story, twenty-terrace building was a masterpiece of modern design, inside and out. He later called it a "medical instrument." Aalto and his wife Aino, also an architect, meticulously co-designed the interior. After interviewing medical staff and patients, they developed everything from door handles that would not catch the sleeve of a doctor's coat to sinks that muffled splashing sounds, to the tables, clocks, lighting fixtures, desks, stools, and chairs. One chair in particular, the austerely sensual bentwood known as the Paimio scroll chair, allowed patients to recline while slim back-slats provided cooling and hand grips helped in getting up. The Paimio chair was so attractive that it was soon imported into the interiors of avant-garde Modernist homes. It was a chair for a clinic, or a house, or part of a machine for health.

At the same time that these two curative Modernist icons were designed and constructed, an unusual home was taking form across the globe on a Los Angeles hillside, the result of another close collaboration between an architect and a doctor—a naturopathic doctor in this case. It would come to be known as the Health House.

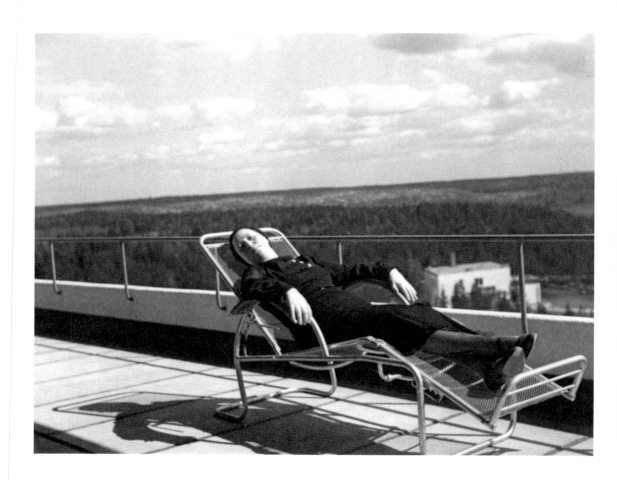

above — **Aino Aalto resting in a chair on the Paimio solarium terrace.**
top right — **Aalto Paimio chairs.**

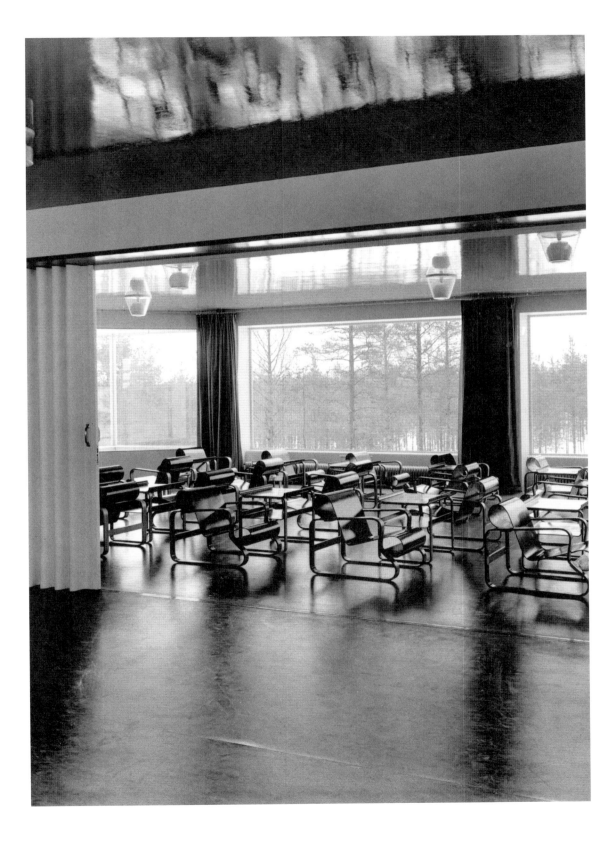

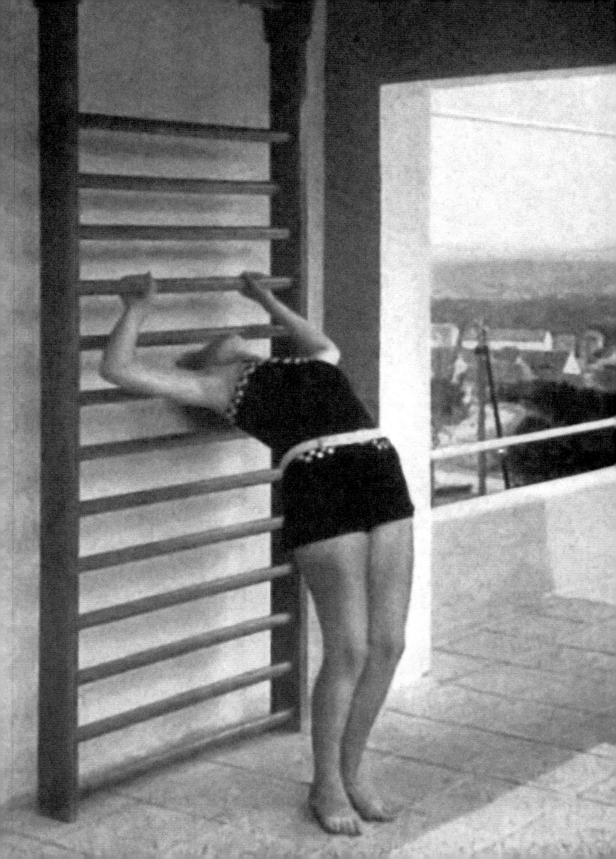

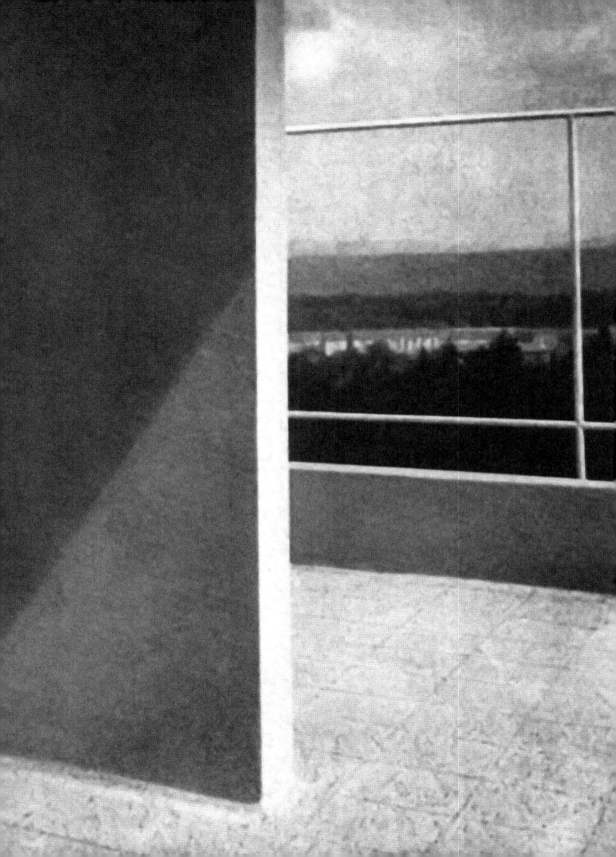

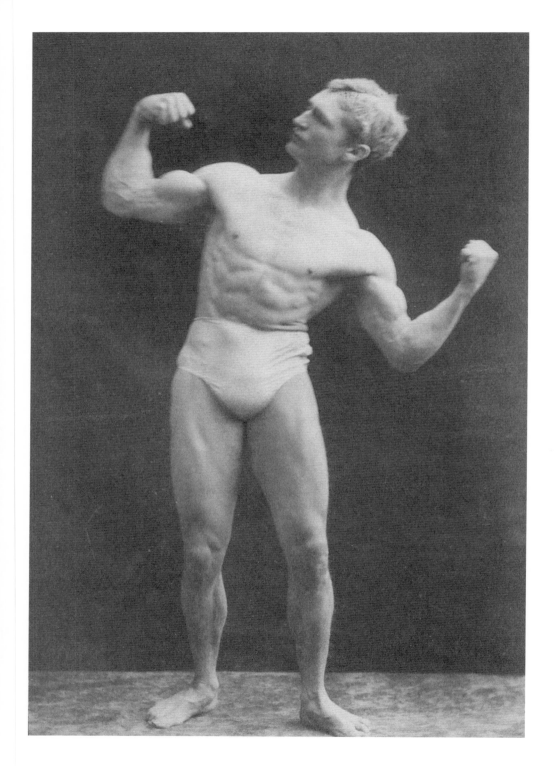

previous page — **A woman exercising on the terrace of Richard Döcker's house in the Werkbundsiedlung, Stuttgart, circa 1926.** above —**Publisher and body builder Bernarr Macfadden.**

THE ARCHITECTS AND THE NATUROPATH

In the fall of 1919, an Austrian architect strolling near the stately Hauptbahnhof train station in Zurich sees a lighted travel poster that grabs his attention. The poster, which would haunt the young man for the next several years, shows an exotic tree rarely seen in Central Europe: a palm. The poster's exact design is unknown but we can imagine it drenched in the sherbet tones of a seaside vignette, all blonde sunshine and aqua waves. The image and its alluring text cast a spell. It read: "CALIFORNIA CALLS YOU." The architect, standing in the cold, blue eyes gazing out from under thick black brows, was named Richard Neutra.

—

Around the same time, in Manhattan, a young upstart named Morris Saperstein pushes into a crowded lecture hall to drink in the rhetoric of Scott Nearing, the radical economist, pacifist, and vocal advocate of vegetarianism. Saperstein was a fan of Nearing and zealously read the speeches and manifestos of his milieu, like Eugene Debs, the labor organizer and Socialist Party presidential candidate, and Upton Sinclair, the journalist and activist from far-away California, who had exposed the vileness of the meatpacking industry.

After the lecture, feeling galvanized, Saperstein may have bought an issue of the popular magazine *Physical Culture* from a newsstand. He admired its charismatic publisher, the famed vegetarian bodybuilder Bernarr Macfadden. The magazine was filled with pulpy tales of physical and mental transformation, promoting Macfadden's homebrewed health evangelism which regularly railed against the sins of doctors, prudery, corsets, physical weakness, and white bread.

Such radical ideas captivated Saperstein. He was raised by Russian Jewish émigré parents in a household that was neither health conscious nor iconoclastic. A typical Saperstein family meal was a heavy affair: brisket, noodles, and cabbage, lacquered in butter. As it turned out, Macfadden's promotion of natural healing, bodily vigor, and no small dose of self-promotion would light an unusual path forward.

—

When Richard Neutra glimpsed the enthralling California travel poster, he was adrift. His nascent architectural career in Vienna had been brutally halted by the First World War. At the age of 22 he was sent to the Balkan trenches. There, like countless others, Neutra became gravely ill, contracting malaria and then a form of tuberculosis. His recovery was slow and his illness (and shifting battle zones) sent him to nearly twenty different hospitals over two years. Upon his final return to Vienna he discovered a city in shambles, suffering from drastic food and housing shortages. Still unwell, he sought recuperation in Switzerland at a small lakeside guesthouse.

At the Swiss border Neutra was able to procure a dish of ham and eggs—a miracle of opulence. He arrived at the guesthouse, an hour outside of Zurich, and began to write inquiries for work in an architecture office. But there was nothing. "Isn't it absurd that a diligent young person cannot find work while the whole world is in need of work?" he lamented in his diary. "Housing shortage and slumbering construction offices—how can it be explained? Listlessly I wander about, without a goal, exhausted. No work, no money, no home, no resting place."

—

Meanwhile in New York, Saperstein attempted to put some of the exhilarating political ideas he'd been hearing about into practice, by organizing a labor walkout at the insurance office where he worked. But too few agents and clerks were willing to stand up to the vocally anti-union management. Discouraged, the headstrong young man quit his job and turned his back on the city, heading west to pursue new horizons and what he likely hoped were broader minds.

Halfway across the country, Saperstein saw an opportunity to explore the natural healing he'd read about in *Physical Culture*. He enrolled at a college in Missouri, probably the one founded by 'magnetic healer' Andrew Taylor Still, a Midwestern doctor well-versed in hydrotherapy, homeopathy, and other nature-cure treatments. It seems that Saperstein soaked it all in. By the time he continued west to launch his career he wielded an arsenal of strong opinions on diet, exercise, and natural cures. Once he reached Los Angeles, Saperstein decided to set down roots. But first he changed his name to Philip M. Lovell—*Dr.* Philip M. Lovell, ND (ND for 'Doctor of Naturopathy'). Legend has it that he saw the benign Anglo surname 'Lovell' on a billboard, added the palatable 'Philip' to it, and like so many others in the young city before and afterward, was reborn.

—

"I wish I could get out of Europe and get to an idyllic tropical island where one does not have to fear the winter, where one does not have to slave but finds time to think, or even more important can have a free spirit," Neutra wrote. Dreaming of escape to sun-drenched liberation, he wrote letters to his Austrian architect friend Rudolph Schindler, living in Los Angeles. Neutra described the impossible obstacles facing architects and construction in postwar Europe and the spiritual bankruptcy of the broken continent. "If only I could get to the United States!" he wrote Schindler. "Could you help me?"

Schindler was a connection to Neutra's life before the war but would also turn out to be a vital link to his future. They had met in Vienna in 1912, a time when the elegant city's avant-garde society of Gustav Klimt, Egon Schiele, Alma Mahler, and Sigmund Freud was in full bloom. The two young friends, at the threshold of their architectural careers, absorbed the new, controversial aesthetic and ideological waves surging through the Austro-Hungarian empire. They both studied with polemical architect Adolf Loos, and would meet at cafés to hear him deliver his Modernist screeds against architectural ornamentation.

Loos was fascinated with the modern industrial Eden that America appeared to be, and repeatedly impressed upon his students that the future lay there. Neutra and Schindler were convinced. This notion was boosted by the first European publication of designs by American architect Frank Lloyd Wright, which captivated architects across the continent. The port-folio had a profound impact, sealing Wright's fame in Europe. Wright's work was defined by the exotic starkness of the Midwestern American plains and a reverence for natural, organic forms stripped down to basic geometry. His vision was fervently embraced as one possible path out of the maze of Europe's dense historicism and fading empires.

"Whoever he was, Frank Lloyd Wright, the man far away, had done something momentous and rich in meaning," wrote Neutra. "This miracle man instilled in me the conviction that, no matter what, I would have to go to the places where he walked and worked." But as it turned out, Schindler was able to make the jour-ney first, in 1914, a few fortunate months before war broke out. Over the next nine years, he wrote Neutra letters of his experiences in the vast, foreign country of America, working for Wright in Chicago and then following him to supervise his projects in Los Angeles. He described a path that Neutra would eventually follow.
—
In 1923 at the age of 28, the newly minted Dr. Lovell opened an office in Downtown Los Angeles advertising himself as a "Drugless Practitioner." While there was a glut of doctors—either drug-pushing or drug-

disdaining —in the area, his business took off, attracting more patients than he could see. Luck was on his side: one of his first patients was Harry Chandler, the powerful publisher of the *Los Angeles Times* newspaper. Chandler had come to Los Angeles to combat tuberculosis, and retained a thirst for natural cures of all stripes. His fondness for Lovell proved profitable.

Lovell was tall, with a strong profile, barrel chest, and bronzed tan. He was not only a popular doctor, but a loquacious one, ever-ready with confident advice. Thanks to his relationship with Chandler, he took over the weekly health column in the *Los Angeles Times* Sunday magazine called "Care of the Body." As it turned out, writing about his beliefs was a natural vocation.

The header of Lovell's column featured a trustworthy, paternal portrait of him from the shoulders up, in a dark suit, tie, and neat, round glasses. His claims may have been eccentric, but he maintained the familiar look of a traditional family doctor. His portrait was bookended by drawings that cheerily illustrated his dietary philosophy: heaps of fruits, vegetables, and leaves. The column itself shared the page with a riot of advertisements for local vegetarian restaurants, doctors, regional sanatoriums, and other salubrious products, from Firmola cream (for sagging chins) to NOK-KA-TAR syrup (for congestion).

Lovell wrote prodigiously, offering sermons, meat-free recipes, and answers to readers' letters on topics that ranged from blisters to gout, childbirth to carrot juice. His tone was pedantic, evangelical, and occasionally condescending; his advice tumbled down from the great temple of health and discipline he claimed to inhabit. At other times he was disarming and good-humored. But Lovell's guru-like desire to share his enlightenment was unflagging. Here he is on sun baths:

"If you have never taken a sun bath, start slowly. Take three minutes the first day, then increase the time two or three minutes daily until you are taking from 20 or 25 minutes to an hour.

Never overheat yourself. The modern solarium should be equipped with a shower. When the body becomes warm or the temperature rises even to a slight degree, get under the shower. If there is no shower, give yourself a cold-water sponge or a simple cold water rub-down.

The sun bath is as precious a part of your daily routine as any bathing hygiene."

On climate cures:

"The ideal environment for one with tuberculosis is the country, especially the dry mountain or desert country where he may bask nude in the sun for hours at a time and where the home environment is such where he may recover his health."

And on fruit candy:

"Grind walnuts, dates, figs and raisins together. Re-grind two or three times. Roll in finely shredded coconut and form in cubes, balls, or any desired shape."

In addition to his column, Dr. Lovell broadcast health talks and an exercise show on a local radio station and delivered well-attended weekly lectures in the auditorium of his Downtown office building. His assistants mailed out free health pamphlets to anyone who requested them. His empire of natural health was thriving.

—

Still in Zurich, Neutra's westward journey remained frustratingly deferred. He had finally found a job at a renowned landscape firm, picking up a refined horticultural education that would serve him well later. He was also introduced to the Niedermanns, a charming, artistic family with four daughters. The youngest pleaded with her mother to "invite the exciting and handsome foreigner" to visit. The eldest, Dione, was an accomplished pianist, cellist, and singer. Upon their meeting Neutra wrote his impressions in his diary: "Dione Niedermann, her legs clad in light blue stockings, looking west." He spent the spring hiking the mountains with the young women and grew close to the whole family.

During this happy reprieve from his troubles, an attraction bloomed between Richard and Dione. Unfortunately, travels for her musical education and for his father's funeral and various temporary jobs kept them separated for a year. They wrote each other almost daily, letters richly marbled with growing affection and sketches of a shared future. "Today I hurried in order to get away at 8:30 to fetch the morning milk," wrote Dione to Richard. "Outside it was foggy and rainy and I needed my heavy boots. One can see our little house from a kilometer's distance. When I was five hundred meters away I saw a white square in the window. Coming nearer, I realized that my family had hung your letter there so I would be sure to see it."

—

In Los Angeles Lovell met and married Leah Press, a progressive teacher whose ideas about child-rearing and healthy living were in sync with his own.[3] A native of Omaha and a graduate of New York University, she was an acolyte of the learn-by-doing educational philosophies of Angelo Patri and John Dewey. When an informal school was formed at a private estate in East Hollywood, Leah was invited to help run it. The land was owned by oil heiress and social progressive

3. They would later co-author the book *Diet for Health by Natural Methods, Together with Health Menus and Recipes: Complete Instructions for the Cure of the Sick Without the Use of Drugs*, published in 1927.

Aline Barnsdall, who had commissioned Frank Lloyd Wright to build her a home, a complex for avant-garde theater, and a school her daughter and other children could attend on a serene hill flecked with olive trees.

"When I met Wright I told him my idea of the ideal school," recalled Leah Lovell. "Little tables for the children which would be separated so each child could work alone, lockers and cupboards four feet high so the children could open the door. All classes outside." At the kindergarten, Leah met another progressive educator, Pauline Schindler (née Gibling), the wife of Rudolph Schindler. The Schindlers had come to Los Angeles at Wright's request for Rudolph to oversee the construction of Barnsdall's complex. Pauline, a fiery composer and social activist who had been living in Chicago, taught with Leah for several years, guiding their own children as well as those of other like-minded families.

A photograph of Leah and Pauline shows an idyllic scene in a sundrenched garden where they are holding hands in a circle with their young students (including two sons of the photographer Edward Weston). Most of the children are barefoot and naked but for underwear. Not surprisingly for the wife of Dr. Lovell, it appears that sunbathing was part of the school's curriculum. "All classes outside," she had told Wright.

It was in this atmosphere, among the small liberal minority whom Pauline later referred to as "those who rejected the idiotic slavery of the public school system," that the Lovells became friends with the Schindlers. The friendship would shape both couples' lives, as well as Neutra's.

—

Now in Berlin, Neutra secured a position in the office of celebrated architect Erich Mendelsohn. Dione was finally able to join him to continue her music studies there. They married and had a baby named Frank, honoring Richard's architectural idol. In spite of these personal gains, Neutra's yearning to leave Europe did not fade. At last, in 1923, he was able to afford passage across the Atlantic.

Neutra pieced together some small jobs in New York and then headed to Chicago, home of new steel skyscrapers and close to his hallowed mentor, Wright. Schindler had told Wright about his talented emigrant friend who yearned to meet him. Perhaps that was enough to warrant an invitation to visit the famously egotistical elder, or perhaps Wright was impressed by Neutra's seriousness, talent, and knowledge of European architecture's postwar developments. Either way, Neutra was offered a rare and coveted opportunity: to live and work with Wright at his home, Taliesin, the stunning compound Neutra likened to "a Japanese temple district," set among the lush, emerald hills of Wisconsin.

"It was like coming into the presence of a unicorn," wrote Neutra of finally meeting his hero. At Taliesin, Neutra's days were spent absorbing Wright's fiery genius, while tranquil evenings centered around the grand hearth, drawing or admiring Wright's collection of Japanese art while Dione, who had joined him there, played cello and sang.

—

Traversing the Hollywood Hills, the Lovells regularly socialized in a small archipelago of bold new homes. There were Wright's buildings for Aline Barnsdall, his house for Leah Lovell's sister Harriet Freeman and her husband, and a house designed, built, and occupied by the Schindlers. The families gathered for their children's lessons, as well as political meetings and artistic salons. Such convergences were not unusual—clients of modern architecture were often progressives who had departed from social norms in one way or another (such as a single mother of means like Barnsdall). There was a strong sense that new ways of living demanded new architecture—and that new architec-

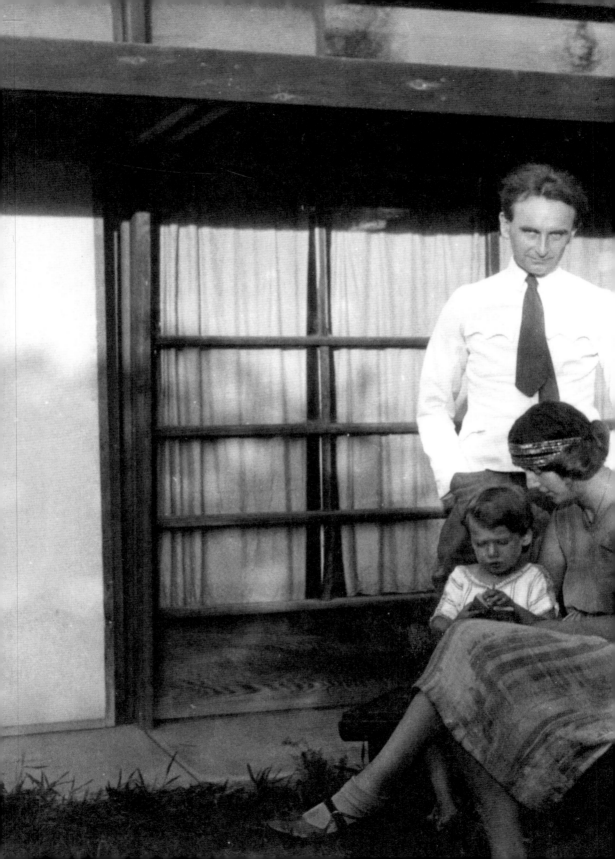

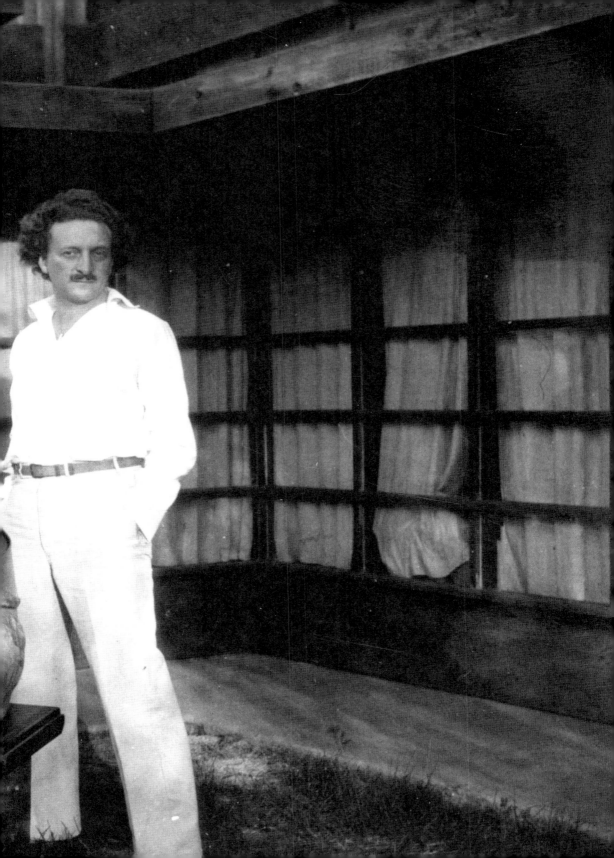

ture would in turn mold a new, improved humanity.

The reverse was likewise believed: old architecture could only reproduce old idioms. Los Angeles, at the time, was full of either replicas of other times and other places, or hastily built structures thrown up to house the constantly booming population. Wright had allegedly once quipped, "Tip the world over on its side and everything loose will land in Los Angeles." He disdained the local housing, claiming "all was flatulent or fraudulent with a cheap opulence. Tawdry Spanish Medievalism was now rampant." The writer Carey McWilliams later deemed the rapid spread of white-walled, red-tiled Spanish-style homes "the stucco rash." Familiar East Coast and Midwest replications mushroomed: brick, peaked roofs, heavy shutters and small rooms. They invoked hidebound traditions better left behind: children learning by dull repetition, pallor, pot roast.

As Lovell grew accustomed to the unusual, austere spaces his friends were building, he paid particular interest to the relationship between domestic space and physical health. This became evident in his "Care of the Body" column. Take, for example, this passage from 1924:

"Besides the value of the outdoor sleeping room as a children's playground, a flat, open roof can be of immense value as a sun parlor. The value of sun bathing for anemia, tuberculosis, and practically all of the wasting diseases has been shown repeatedly. An open roof with a view-tight fence solves this problem without offense to the neighbors. There, for several hours per day, the children may play nude in the healthful sunshine. There the sick and the suffering may get the benefit of life-giving rays of the sun without the expense of the sanatorium. There man may get in touch with the cosmic forces of nature far better than in closed rooms and confined spaces."

previous page — Richard Neutra, R.M. Schindler, Dione Neutra, and Dion Neutra, at the Kings Road house they briefly shared, West Hollywood, California.

Healthful housing soon became a regular feature of Lovell's writing. "When we consider that we spend at least half of each day's hours in the home, the importance of building a structure for health purposes is evident," he noted. "In the past, such elements as beauty, convenience, and comfort have played the dominant parts. Houses for health are even yet relatively unknown." He noted how difficult it was to find an architect or builder who understood "fundamental health principles."

—

A letter composed in one of these pioneering Los Angeles houses was mailed to Neutra at Taliesin during the frigid Wisconsin winter of 1925. It was from Schindler, who wrote, "I would be very pleased to receive you here and help you over the initial difficulties, as far as it is in my power." He added wryly, "We shall not starve." During the war and its aftermath, Schindler's letters had delivered scenes of exotic lands, tales of tempestuous experiences working for Wright, and a sense of boundless architectural opportunity. "I am overjoyed when a letter arrives from you," Neutra had written. Their years of correspondence were bearing fruit.

While the atmosphere at Taliesin was enchanting, the work was unreliable and sometimes unpaid. Wright was notoriously difficult, clashing with his clients and forbidding his employees to work on their own designs even during their free time. Neutra felt ready to strike out on his own. In February, he and his family set out for Los Angeles by train and were warmly invited to rent half of the two-family house that Schindler had built a few years earlier. Once they arrived, Dione called the house "strange... which has its own beauty considering how little money [Schindler] has."

Rising from a field of grass in West Hollywood, on a street named Kings Road, Schindler's low-slung house of gray concrete and rich redwood was designed with his and his wife Pauline's social ideals in mind. The house accommodated two couples, with communal kitchen and living spaces. Each resident, male and female, would have their own studio. Japanese-style screens and sliding doors opened the house up to the yard, while hedges divided the outdoor spaces into intimate rooms.

Soon after the Schindlers first came to California in 1920, they went camping for several weeks in Yosemite National Park. Their exposure to the elements, where nature and shelter were divided by a simple flap of canvas cloth, proved influential. Describing his house, Schindler explained, "The theme fulfills the basic requirements of a camper's shelter. [Each room has] a protected back, an open front, a fireplace and a roof." Passersby must have been baffled by the alien structure, and by its residents.

In his Mexican huaraches, open-collared silk shirts, and the tousled dark hair he cut himself, Schindler was the image of a freethinking artist. Wright had called him "an incorrigible bohemian." Pauline wore loose linen caftans, little makeup, and wielded strong opinions. Their Kings Road house—indoors and out—became a center for lively Sunday gatherings with a close circle of agitators, artists, poets, dancers, composers, and socialists. Concerts and dance performances were staged beneath the stars as wind shivered through the bamboo groves. Intimate readings took place in the glow of the rough-hewn fireplaces, the flames reflected in copper hoods, shadows cast on the walls. Schindler had created a proto-modern, primeval setting, a style of architecture he claimed was "as Californian as the Parthenon is Greek and the Forum Roman." His integration of natural materials and outdoor space was "the beginning of a new 'classic' growth drinking California sap."

"The climate suits me here just fine!" Dione wrote to her mother in Switzerland. "I cannot remember when I felt so well anywhere else." The idyllic climate and bohemian lifestyle at Kings Road loosened her hard-working husband as well; soon Richard was sunbathing around the yard and donning only bathing trunks as he sketched, read, and wrote. Everyone slept outdoors on the flat rooftop porches (or 'sleeping baskets' as Schindler called them). Richard wrote of glancing "from my sleeping porch into the green spring greenery. It has rained yesterday and this night. The leaves of our trumpet vine glisten with raindrops. The huge bamboo stalks—together with a contingent of birds, who, with their twittering, apply the colorful background music of Dione's songs, sway gently in the breeze."

The two architects, separated for so long, began collaborating on drawings and plans. They made quite a splash in Los Angeles with their Austrian accents, unusual dress, and twin cars. But clients for their vanguard styles weren't easy to find. Most people wanted fast, cheap, and familiar. The stucco rash reigned.

In the wake of his interest in hygienic homes, Lovell had invited Schindler to contribute an architect's perspective to his weekly newspaper column. In six installments, Schindler discussed practical matters of interest to the everyday homeowner interested in health—like ventilation, plumbing, and furniture. But the topics were couched within a philosophical, almost mystical context: small windows, for example, became a symbol of primitive man's fear and suspicion.

Schindler's vehemence about the need for new architecture matched the doctor's fervor for healthful living. As Lovell preached to "heed nature's slightest warning," Schindler railed against the uselessness of basements and chandeliers, which he excoriated as "'ornamental' atrocities with imitation candles." He

87

prophesied the following, clearly based on his Kings Road house:

"The house and the dress of the future will give us control of our environment, without interfering with our mental and physical nakedness. Our rooms will descend close to the ground and the garden will become an integral part of the house. The distinction between the indoors and the out-of-doors will disappear. The walls will be few, thin, and removable... [we] will sleep in the open."

When the Lovells had decided to commission their own avant-garde dwellings in the early 1920s, wrought in the service of healthful ideology, Schindler was their natural choice. (As Lovell declared, underscoring his self-perception as an enlightened free-thinker, "I was not going to build my house the same as the woman from Peoria!" [a provincial town in Illinois]). They hired Schindler to build three unusual vacation houses, each in natural settings driving distance from the city—in the mountains, the desert, and by the coast. The desert house burned down (through no fault of Schindler's), and the mountain cabin's roof collapsed under the first heavy snow. But Schindler's masterful and pioneering house in Newport Beach, south of Los Angeles, remains. Employing new materials and unusual forms, the angular concrete house, completed in 1926, expressed the doctor's ethos with a dramatic open-air sunbathing and sleeping porch facing the gleaming Pacific waves.

The Lovells and their growing family (they would have three sons) enjoyed the beach house, but they also wanted a mainstay in the city, closer to Philip's Downtown office. They began looking at sites in the hilly area of Los Feliz and thinking about possible designs. While Schindler had a deep understanding of their values, his experimental buildings always went over budget and hadn't functioned well. Meanwhile,

right — The Lovell Beach House, Newport Beach, California.

the Lovells had gotten to know the other intriguing Viennese architect recently arrived at the Kings Road house.

Neutra and Schindler had similar backgrounds and mentors. But as they learned after trying to collaborate, their styles, temperaments, and work habits differed greatly. Schindler was a consummate and intuitive artist, whereas Neutra had a more disciplined bent. Schindler was inspired by earthy notions of the cave and the tang of sticky California sap, while Neutra had absorbed nine more years of an evolving European Modernism that espoused a rationalistic, machine aesthetic. For Neutra, a building could only be considered 'modern' if it took full advantage of industrial technology. What might *he* design for the naturopath?

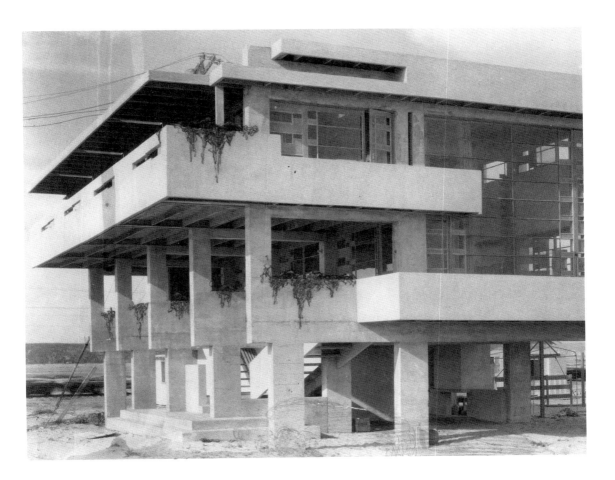

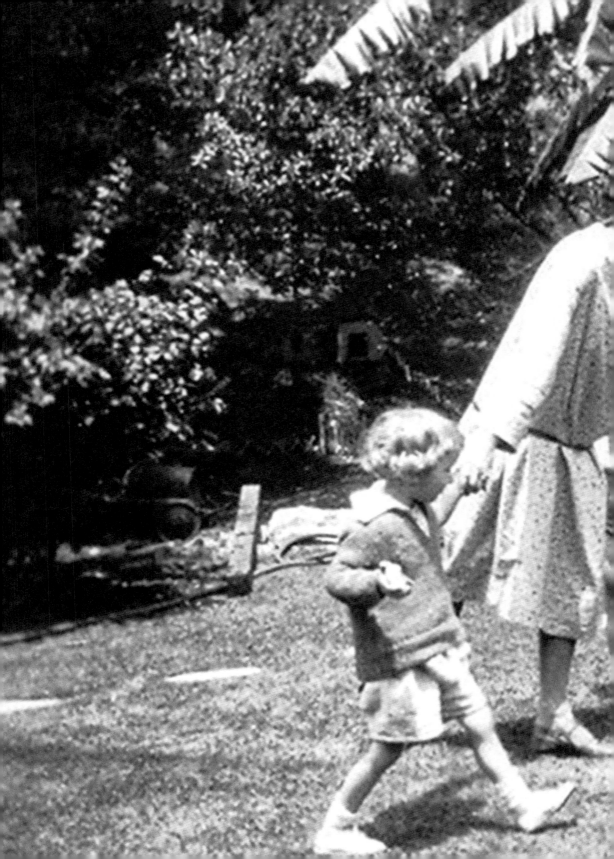

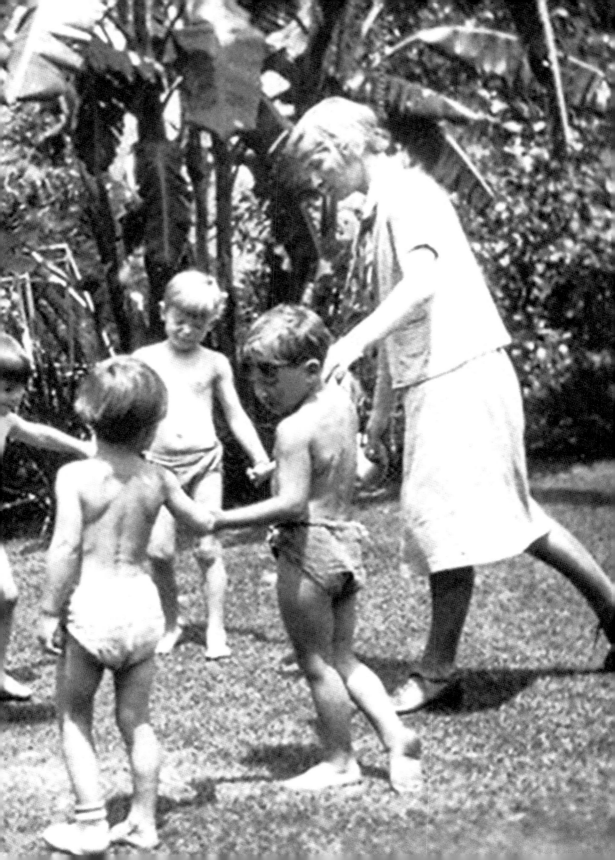

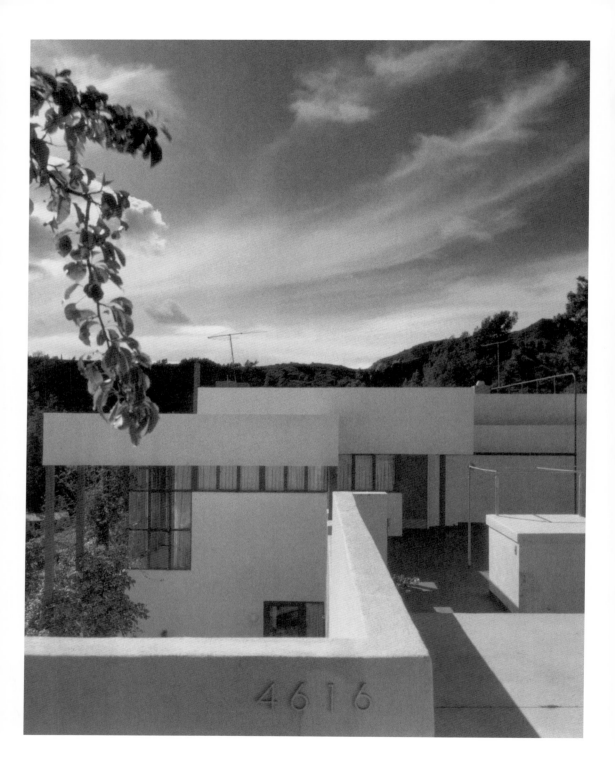

92 previous page — Pauline Schindler, Leah Lovell, and children in Leah's "School in the Garden," Argyle Avenue, Hollywood, California, circa 1925. above — View of the Health House, located at 4616 Dundee Drive, Los Angeles, California.

THE HEALTH HOUSE

Over several weekends in December 1929, thousands of curious Los Angeles residents traversed the winding, chaparral-fringed roads near Griffith Park to tour an extraordinary new house. They were not coming to gawk at the mansion of a film star, or to peer behind the heavy doors of the lavish Tudor manors, Italianate villas, or red-tiled Spanish haçiendas built for the city's wealthiest. They were answering the call of the popular, charismatic Dr. Philip Lovell, who had personally invited them, via the pages of the *Los Angeles Times*:

"For years I have periodically written articles telling you how to build your home so that you can derive from it the maximum degree of health and beauty service. I have written on miscellaneous problems such as lighting, heating, hydrotherapy equipment, labor-saving devices, sleeping porches, material for construction and other health features. Always at the end of each article was the thought, 'If I ever build a home myself'—At last the day has arrived."

His column listed the street address as the terminal cul-de-sac of Dundee Drive (eastward over the hills from the Hollywood sign). It also provided a drawn map and announced open hours to visit his "newly constructed home built for health." Each day, he noted, his architect Richard Neutra would give a guided tour at three in the afternoon. On the appointed weekends, Dundee Drive was lined bumper-to-bumper with cars, their curvaceous, beetle-like forms and wooden-spoked wheels contrasting with the sharply-angled white modern house. As the thousands of visitors poured in, their reactions were startled and confused. "Moon architecture!" exclaimed someone overheard by Neutra, who was undoubtedly eavesdropping. A more accurate description would have been sun architecture.

93

Built on a steep incline, the house consisted of several rectangular slabs cascading down the hillside in sleek interlocking layers: white, glass, white, glass. Suspended porches and overhangs jutted out or wrapped around flatly, like trays for catching sunlight. Inside, the rooms were painted a reserved palette of white, black, grey, and blue. The house incorporated many tropes of European Modernism that Neutra had absorbed and mastered, but its setting was radically different. The walls of windows framed views of mostly empty wild hills, where coyotes might be glimpsed loping through the brush.

A revolutionary technology enabled the house's translucent quality—a structural skeleton of thin steel. Local contractors had worked with iron and wood frames, but never steel, so Neutra acted as head contractor as well as designer. He recalled standing in the darkness before morning broke at the site, where tons of steel lay waiting to be put together, "to check every one of the thousand pre-punched bolt holes and shop-cut coverplates." As the sun rose, the Lovells and a group of representatives from the Bethlehem Steel Corporation watched as Neutra began to oversee the assembly of the massive frame. A mere forty hours later the scaffolding was up, glinting on the hillside— an unprecedented sight. It was the first steel-framed house in the United States.

Once the frame was complete, Neutra utilized a relatively new technique to shoot concrete from a 250-foot pneumatic hose onto a skin of mesh, casting a thin hard shell around the frame. When Wright heard about what Neutra was working on, he wrote him a letter saying, "The boys tell me you are building a building of steel for [a] residence—which is really good news. Ideas like that one are what this poor fool country needs to learn from Corbusier, Stevens, Oud, and Gropius. I am glad you're the one to 'teach' them."

right —Views of the Health House pool deck.

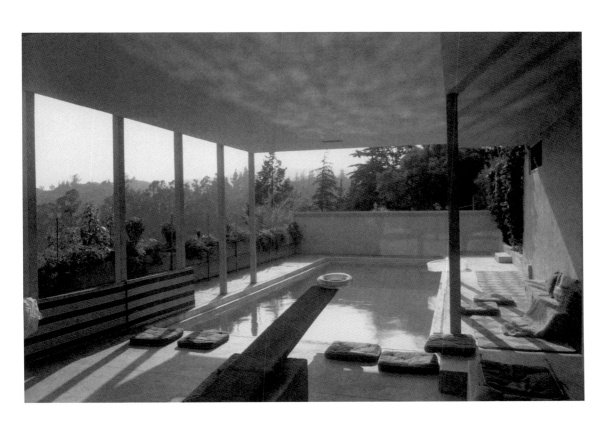

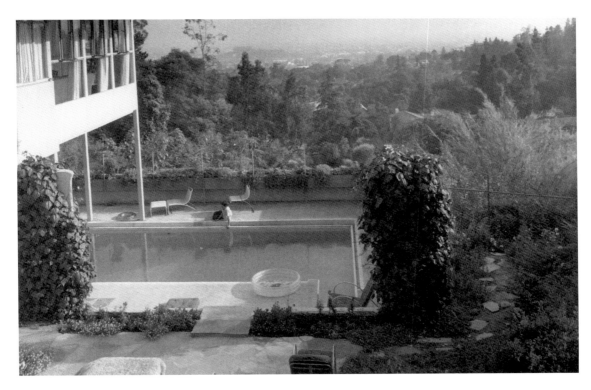

Lovell, ever the ringmaster, went on to describe the unique amenities of his home for those of his readers who would be unable to make the visit up the hillside.

"There are plenty of opportunities throughout the house for nude sun baths privately taken for each member. Many of the windows are of the latest invention of glass, admitting ultra-violet light. The bathrooms are completely equipped with hydrotherapy equipment, including such things as sitz baths, multiple marathon showers, and the latest type of sanitary fixtures... The ventilation, sunshine, and light ideas are exceedingly modern... every inside bedroom has its accompanying sleeping porch so that sleeping can be done outdoors."

Neutra had spent a year collecting information from each member of the family, including their cook, Mrs. Westerman, about daily habits and domestic needs. The kitchen was equipped with modern time-saving conveniences "interesting to every practical house-wife," and was designed for the preparation of his family's vegetarian—often raw—diet. The hillside slopes were planted with an orchard, including one hundred avocado trees. Rare for the time, the house boasted its own backyard swimming pool (for laps and sunning, certainly not for the dietary sins of barbecues and cocktail parties). Lovell, ever averse to synthetic chemicals, was "violently opposed to chlorine," so he devised a method of recycling the chemical-free pool water every two weeks to douse the hillside, then refilled the pool with a hose.

The outdoor spaces emphasized exercise and move-ment, especially for the children, with a playground, a wading pond "where they can sail their boats and grow their fish," an outdoor schoolroom (which Leah Lovell would expertly oversee) with areas for carpentry and clay work, a basketball and handball court, and gymnastic equipment. Lovell noted that the house possessed "many of the features which schools should have, but most of them do not." He described the entire house and grounds as being, for their three sons, "a social school in which they will learn their life habits." If architecture shapes its inhabitants, children, unmarked and malleable, would benefit the most from this improved way of living. Lovell hoped it would introduce "a modern type of architecture and establish it firmly in California, where new and individualistic architecture is necessary."

In describing the house, Neutra pronounced the "light, airy skeleton, partitioned off... by thin, well-insulating membranes" as the "prototype of the progressive building." It needed no false ornamentation because it was adorned with natural vegetation. Here, austere European Modernism fused with the fertile Californian landscape. Neutra concluded that the house, with its outdoor sleeping porches and dining areas, sounded the dominant note of "today's inclination for the out-of-doors," necessitating new forms, structures, and technical details. It was a "machine in the garden."

This phrase, offered by architectural historian Thomas Hines, alludes to the mechanic, scientific, or futuristic building in harmony with its natural surroundings. It was a feature common to many of the architectural projects that would come to be called California Modernism. At the Health House, the embrace of nature was defined by the lightest and most invisible separation, enabled by new uses of steel and glass. And despite the house's setting among untamed mountains and thickets of wild sage, Neutra mounted the headlights of a Model T Ford into the wall of the main interior stairway, a nod to the efficiency and rationalism of his health machine.

After the doors were closed, and the gawking public drove back down the hill, life at the Lovell Health House continued more or less as he'd planned. The

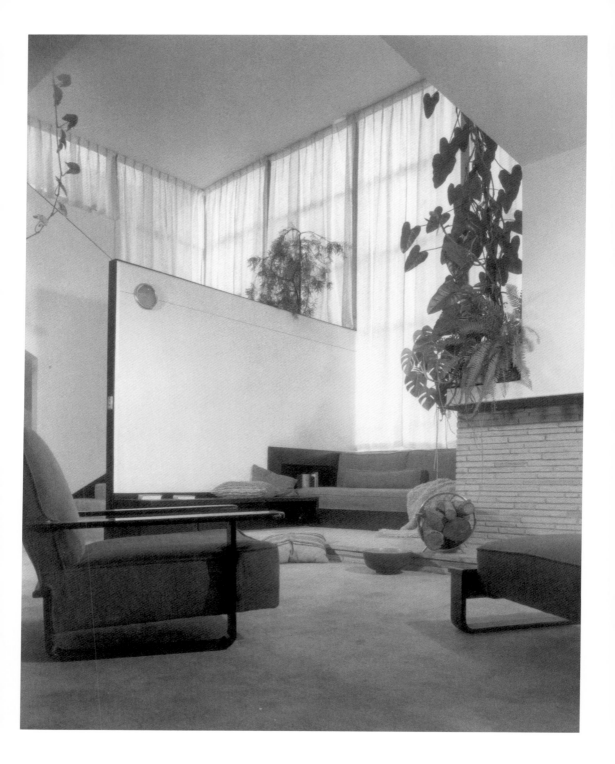

Inside the Health House.

doctor and his family swam in the pool, cultivated therapeutic tans, and consumed their homemade fruit juices and crudités. The boys grew strong and lithe using the outdoor exercise equipment, and according to their father enjoyed excellent health. Lovell later boasted that there was "never a drug or doctor [other than himself] in the house." The house, it seemed, was medicine enough.

—

In a letter to Neutra many years later, in the entirely different—but familiar—culture of 1969, Lovell wrote: "Richard, you and RMS [Schindler] were the 'Hippies', the protesters of those years in the field of architecture—and I was the master 'Hippy' of my forte, not believing in the 'Establishment' of orthodox medicine, and most other things pertinent to the 'Establishment' of those days." Indeed the three men's willingness to experiment with unorthodox ways of living was certainly rare for their era, some forty years before the term 'hippie' was widely known.

The Health House launched Neutra's name into architectural circles around the world, and it became a mainstay in the exhibitions, periodicals, and books that shaped and defined Modernism throughout the 1930s and into the mid-twentieth century. He marveled, "How could I have proceeded from such obscurity and a starvation diet to something like a career?" He went on to build many more projects in Los Angeles and abroad, including the most ultra-Californian of building types: a drive-in church with an indoor/outdoor pulpit facing both pews and parking lot.

Neutra's style evolved over the years, but a focus on the health-giving elements of design was often evident. (And not only in design: Dione recalled that spending a lot of time with the Lovell family had caused them to stop drinking coffee and eat more fresh fruits and vegetables.) As Neutra later reflected:

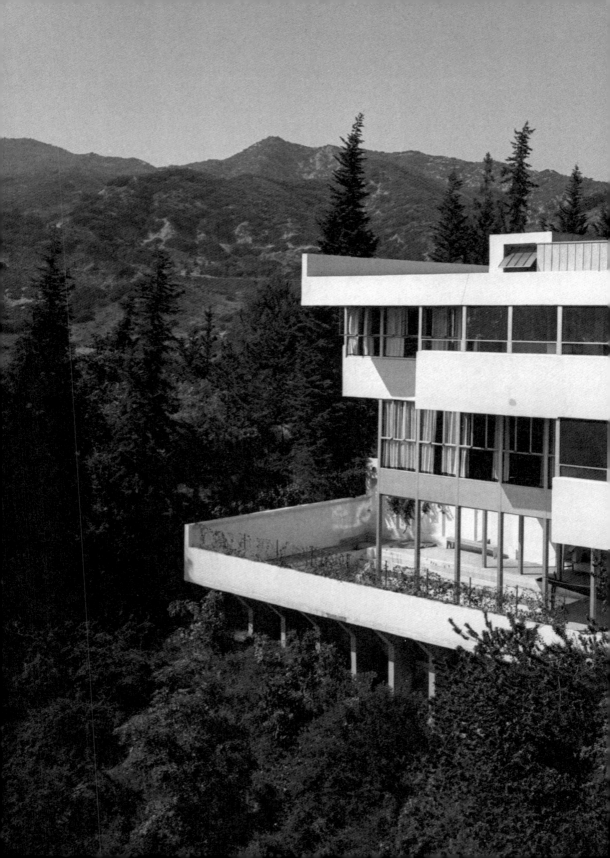

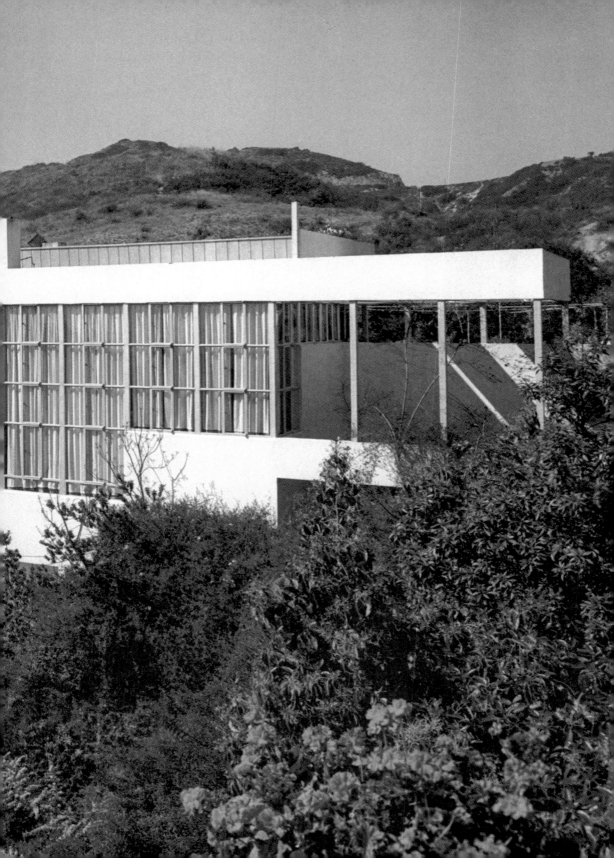

*"The climate of California, at least in those halcyon days
before the citrus groves and bean fields were crowded out
by freeways, parking lots, and subdivisions, was conducive to the germination of a fundamentally fresh form of
architectural growth... I saw that buildings agleam with the
materials of our own time might fraternize with the soil and
psyche of this yet-unspoiled region. This was as important
for the cultivation of our innermost well-being as a sensible
diet and regular exercise, and this was a connection that I
felt I could get across in such a health-conscious climate."*

Nudism also found an advocate in Neutra. In a
little-known article published in 1962 titled 'The
Complex of Nudism,' he addressed the readers of the
recently launched American lifestyle magazine *Nude
Living* about the naturalness of nudity among all
animals, the artifice of clothing and hair dye, and the
importance of nudity to the free expression of human
sexuality. While he didn't discuss architecture explicitly, his musings on the simple, sincere practice of
nudism resonated with the Modernist spirit of paring
forms down to their naked cores.[4]

One of Neutra's apprentices, recalling the early
years of his mentor's work in Los Angeles, playfully
deemed the style "raw-food architecture." The purist
virtues of carrot sticks, palm dates, and coconut oil
were made manifest in his austere, sun-drenched
planes of radiant health. No extra adornments were
necessary. Critic Esther McCoy built on the sobriquet,
noting, "The 'raw-food architecture' of the 20s became
the caviar by mid-century." In other words the pioneering indoor-outdoor homes evolved, rather quickly,
into status symbols.[5] In the new era of antibiotics,
the medicinal aura of a healthful, sun-trapping house
was translated into other symbols: leisure, pleasure,
wealth, the good life. The Hollywood Hills were soon
dotted with flat-roofed modern homes whose walls of

102

glass, turquoise pools, and austere patios hung over the glittering spread of the city below.

Meanwhile Lovell continued expanding his crusade. Two years after moving into his futuristic house of hygiene, he decided to travel to the Soviet Union—still his perceived center of political utopia—to introduce his comrades to the avocado. He had long recommended the buttery fruit as a primary source of healthful fats and wanted to bring his gospel to the site of the world's great social revolution. But the trip was not the glorious exchange Lovell had imagined. First, the avocado seeds were seized by German authorities, who thought they might be explosives. Once cleared, he left for Moscow to meet with the Minister of Agriculture but received only a lukewarm, distracted reception. Dismayed, he tried to leave the country, except he was robbed of his wallet, passport, and pants while sleeping on a Kiev-bound train. Eventually, after appealing to the embassy, he got out, greatly disillusioned. Lovell spent the rest of his years back in California, dispensing health advice and living, naturally, into his 80s.

As for the Health House itself, like its Modernist sisters in Europe, Paimio and Zonnestraal, it still stands. It is a relic, now, to a time when cures were built with steel and glass.

4. Neutra's secretary, an ardent nudist and nude-yoga practitioner who arranged the interview for the magazine, was profiled in the same issue, nude, as "Audre: Able and Agile." As historian Sarah Schrank has noted, the link between nudism and modern architecture had also been mocked by more traditional, or indeed conservative, detractors. For example, architect Leicester B. Holland's diatribe in the March 1937 issue of *The Architect and Engineer* magazine: "the Nudist costume has much in common with modern architecture; it is functional, it eschews all ornament, it revels in sunlight… All things considered, I am convinced that Nudist and modern architecture do or should go hand in hand… Nudism in its philosophy is the negation of ornament, the negation of artificiality, and therefore, I believe, the negation of man's pride in his humanity as distinguished from simple animal nature." He concludes, rather brazenly, "It is the negation of civilization."

5. Three of Neutra's apprentices helped carry the wave forward with commissions to build the now-iconic Case Study Houses in Los Angeles after the Second World War. The utopian project, commissioned by the avant-garde *Arts & Architecture* magazine, aimed to create affordable, replicable modern homes to address the postwar housing shortage. Instead, the spectacular prototypes became one-of-a-kind covetable landmarks.

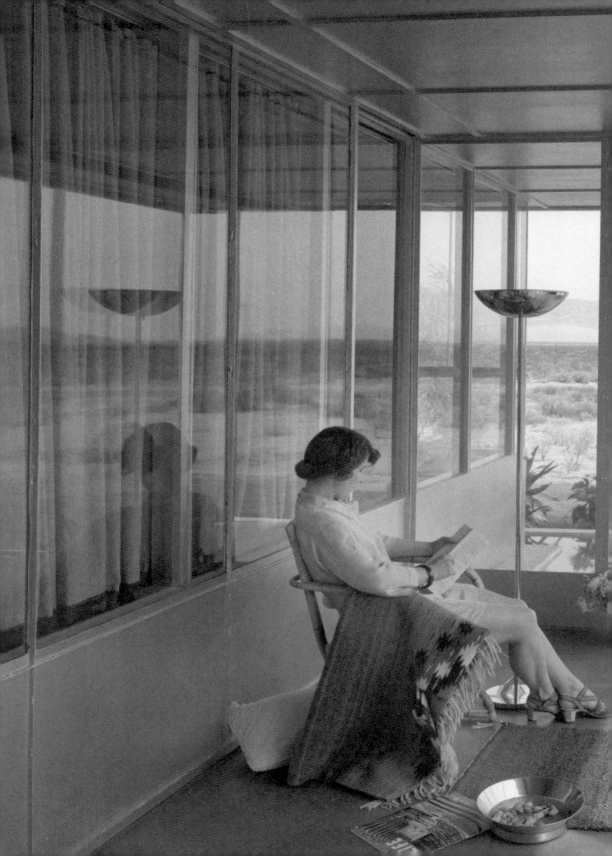

I n the winter of 1936 Grace Lewis Miller piled her two young children into the car in St. Louis, Missouri, and drove to California. She was heading for Palm Springs, a small desert city that had grown affluent and become glamorous as a resort for Hollywood movie stars. It seemed a safe bet in the middle of the Depression. Recently widowed, Miller sought to build a modern but modest winter house with a studio for teaching the Mensendieck system of exercise.

Dr. Bess Mensendieck, an American, studied medicine, posture, and kinesthesiology in Zurich at the turn of the last century, becoming one of the first female physicians to qualify in Europe. Her first book, *Korperkultur der Frau*, was published in Germany in 1905, and featured a women's exercise system of 53 economical movements for the "body machine," demonstrated nude. She believed the entire body, and the spirit, could be restored through these natural, efficient movements. Historian Stephen Leet describes a Mensendieck instructor as "playing the multiple roles of body architect/sculptor/therapist."

It was during a trip to Sweden in 1930 that Miller first encountered the Mensendieck system. She had also visited a major exhibition of new modern architecture on the trip. The two innovative ideas, both concerned with the pared-down beauty inherent in functionality, apparently became intertwined in her mind, and she trained to become a certified instructor of the Mensendieck system. After she had completed her training, she opened a studio in St. Louis, where a local newspaper deemed her "a professor of body mechanics."

Miller had read about Richard Neutra's work in architecture magazines, learning how his Health House blended a Modernist vocabulary with the California landscape. She called him and explained her needs. It was a small commission for him but it seems he was partly drawn in by the challenge of designing, again, towards a therapeutic purpose. Neutra already knew of the Mensendieck system due to its popularity in Central and Northern Europe, and he asked that the house be named "Mensendieck House."

Miller, as an architect of the body, and Neutra, as architect of her house and studio, collaborated closely in the design process. She requested a studio for students wearing a "minimum of clothing," northern light "as in a sculptor's studio," a mirrored wall and a curtain that could be drawn during lessons and retracted at other times to extend the living room seamlessly. The austere result has been likened to a Japanese tea house (Neutra had visited Japan in 1930). The experience of seamlessness continued through to the house's many broad windows and strategically placed mirrors, exhibiting and doubling the vast desert landscape. Glass bedroom doors opened directly outdoors and a screened-in porch extended the living space outside as well. As Miller noted, "all the spaces indoors should be part of the spaces outdoors. There are canyons and snow-covered mountains immediately to the west and the wide desert to the south and east... I wanted this house to be a part of this setting." The low-slung building was clad in pale cement, flat roof overhangs provided shade, and a square pool threw patterns of light onto the ceiling. At night the sparsely furnished house seemed almost translucent, glowing like a lantern.

As Leet has noted, Grace Miller's house was one of only two modernist homes built for female clients with a focused interest in health during this period. (The other was Marcel Breuer's 1930 Berlin apartment/fitness studio for gymnastics instructor Hilde Levi.) When completed, the house was celebrated in the architecture community, winning several awards and enthusiastic coverage in magazines and journals. However, whether due to the poor economy, competing fitness trends, or a perception that the Mensendieck method was too foreign, Miller failed to attract the Palm Springs clientele she had hoped for. Unable to afford the upkeep of the building, she rented it out during the war. When she returned a few years later she found the house full of dust, scorpions and black widow spiders. The simple, all but translucent structure was so near to nature that the environment had seemingly passed through its walls.

continued from overleaf — **Grace Miller in her home, Palm Springs, California, circa 1937.**

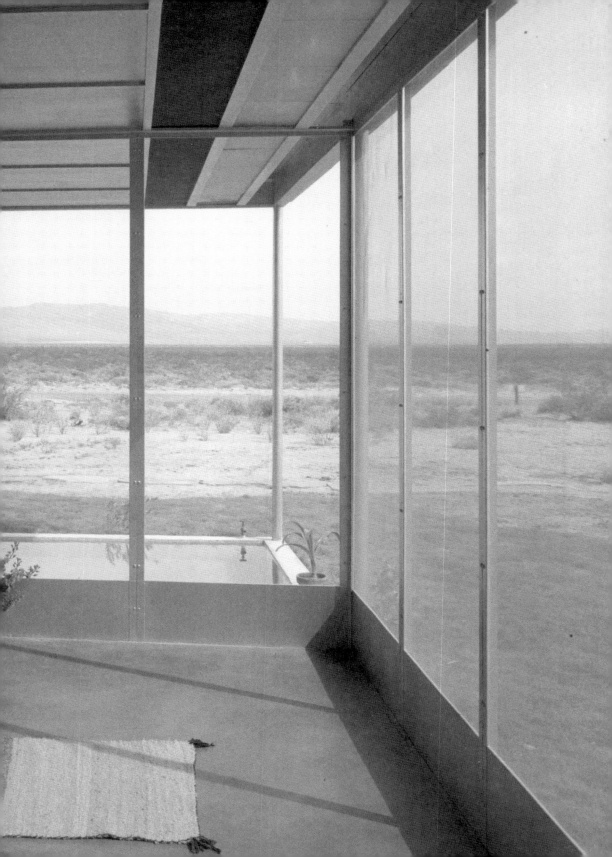

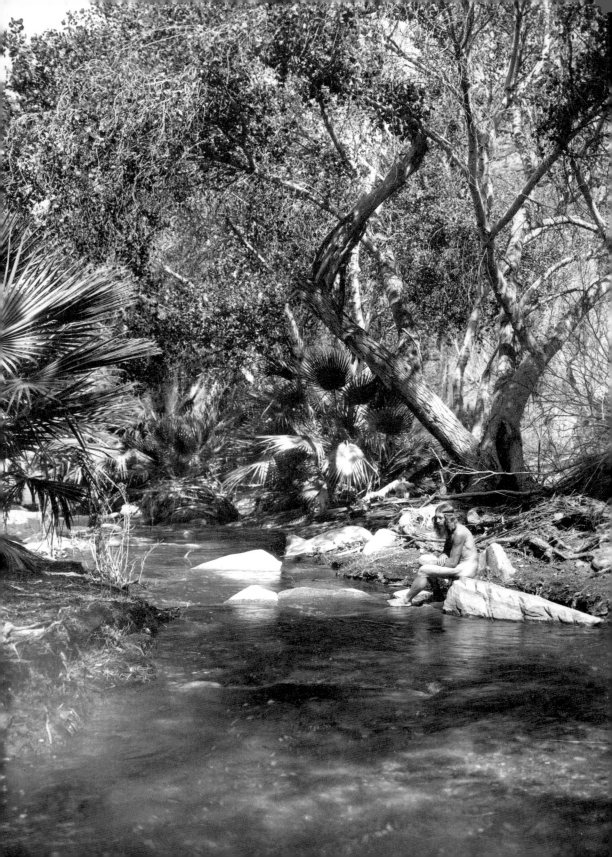

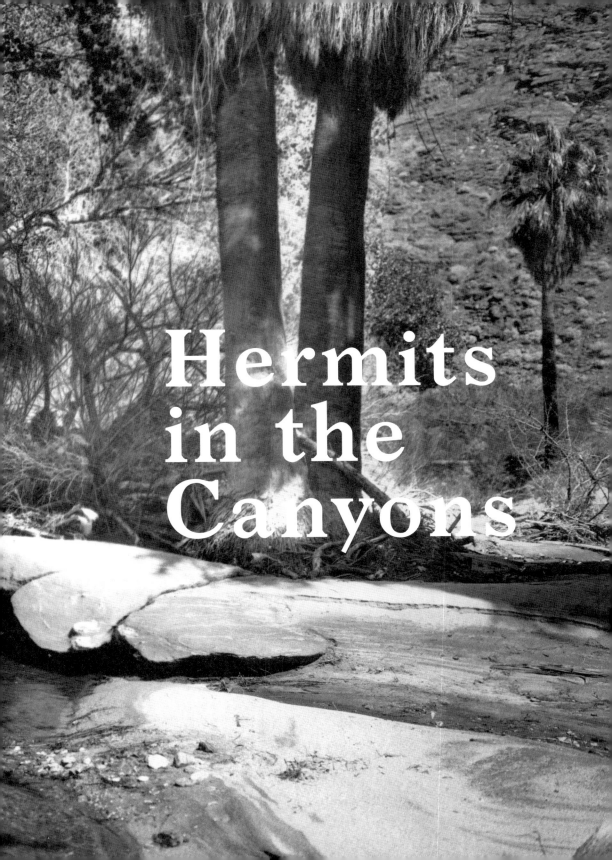

There was a boy
A very strange, enchanted boy
They say he wandered very far
Very far, over land and sea
A little shy and sad of eye
But very wise was he

"Nature Boy," eden ahbez

previous page — **William Pester, the Hermit of Palm Springs, near a stream, circa 1924.**

Sometime after 1906, a strange figure arrived in the desert east of Los Angeles. Seeking an isolated place to settle he found a lush canyon hidden within the folds of bare, reddish-brown mountains, where a natural spring formed a long winding band of green. Hundreds of palm trees grew along the reed-lined stream, sheathed in thick blonde beards of fronds that cascaded to the damp ground. The man set to work gathering palm wood and fronds to build a small hut. Lean, long-haired, and richly bearded himself, this pale-eyed stranger wore homemade sandals and often nothing else. The canyon was home to coyotes, mule deer, quail, and lizards, but he ate no meat. Eventually known as the 'Hermit of Palm Canyon,' William Pester had fled civilization to cultivate a solitary Eden. He had come a very long way.

Other than the sound of dry winds in the fronds and the thrumming and chirping of birds, the canyon was enveloped in a profound silence. Away from the muddy banks and cool canopy of shade, a harsh, crystalline sunlight pounded every surface. The jagged horizon of the brown San Jacinto Mountains vibrated against blue sky. At night a million stars blazed. For over 2,000 years, the Agua Caliente band of the Cahuilla tribe lived in or traveled to such oases to escape the summer heat, which can hit 120 degrees. They gathered water and harvested clusters of black, bead-like fruits from the palms. When Pester arrived on their reservation, he was the only white man among them.

Born Friedrich Wilhelm Pester in a coal-mining town near Leipzig, Germany, in 1885, he left his country around the age of nineteen to escape compulsory military service. Pester crossed Europe, the Atlantic, and the United States alone, working as a laborer. We don't know how he chose this part of California's deserts, but it offered an alien landscape as different from respectable civic life in Germany as could be imagined. As an early settler recounted, the Mexico-bound train stopped in the middle of the night at the 'station,' which consisted of a water tank and a small, white, hand-painted sign that read "Palm Springs." Pester later told a journalist that he came to California to "study himself with untrammeled nature as his classroom."

Pester spent his days simply, foraging for food, bathing in a crude bath he dug out of a natural spring, strumming his slide guitar, and exploring the canyons and rocky hills among barrel-shaped cacti and skeletal, silver-green creosote brush. His meandering walks echoed the movements of local health seekers in the region who pursued the cure of sundrenched outdoor exercise. But Pester's ideas about what needed to be cured were altogether different.

"All man's troubles, sickness, anxieties, and discontent, come from a departure from nature," he once explained. "I was never sick, because I obey the laws of nature and my food is simple... I have little use for money, and I am not bothered by politics or religion, as I have no special creed." Pester had struck out to cultivate a solitary life in tune with nature. He described it as returning to the Garden of Eden.

Palm Springs, some 8 miles from his canyon, was growing from a scattering of shacks into a small town. Its main boarding house, which had once welcomed visitors with pulmonary ailments, was converted into a reputable resort for pleasure-seeking tourists. To his dismay, Pester became one of the desert's attractions. He may have fled civilization, but civilization would not let him go. On September 9, 1916, the *Los Angeles Times* ran a nearly full-page photograph of the long-haired Pester squatting by his palm cabin. "Hermit's Cabin Built of Palms Near Palm Springs," the headline barked. In the picture, ten tourists are standing near him, looking overdressed in their white tailored clothes and clean hats. Soon, the perilous dirt road leading to his cabin was lined with Model T Fords on weekends.

"There are too many people here now," Pester told a journalist in 1922. "When I first came to Palm Springs there were only a few Indians and an occasional white man. Now there are tourists all the time and motion-picture people pestering me and I am no longer able to lead the life of contemplation that I desire." The stream of visitors caused him to announce plans to leave for a more remote location in southern Mexico.

But he ended up staying. Despite his annoyance, he realized the visitors were curious about his unusual lifestyle and might be open to his beliefs. Seeing how interested they were in photographing him, Pester began producing postcards for sale. On one side, black-and-white images depict his ruggedly exotic visage, posing with beatific calm. On the back he printed his life doctrines about the laws of nature: "Eat fresh fruits and vegetables, take sunbaths, drink pure water, and abstain from unnatural stimulants like alcohol and caffeine." Between postcard sales and charging for telescope views of the moon, Pester was able to sustain his humble diet of fruit and bread and even purchase some land away from tourists' eyes, where he eventually planted an orchard of citrus, date, and nut trees. He remained a desert legend, a vision of possibility to others seeking a return to nature.

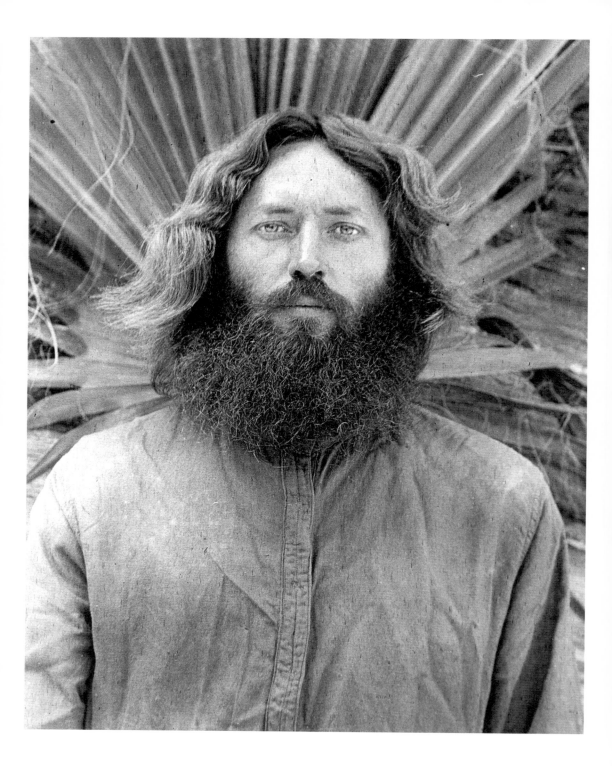

114   above —Portrait of William Pester. right — Post card of William Pester, the 'Nature Man.'

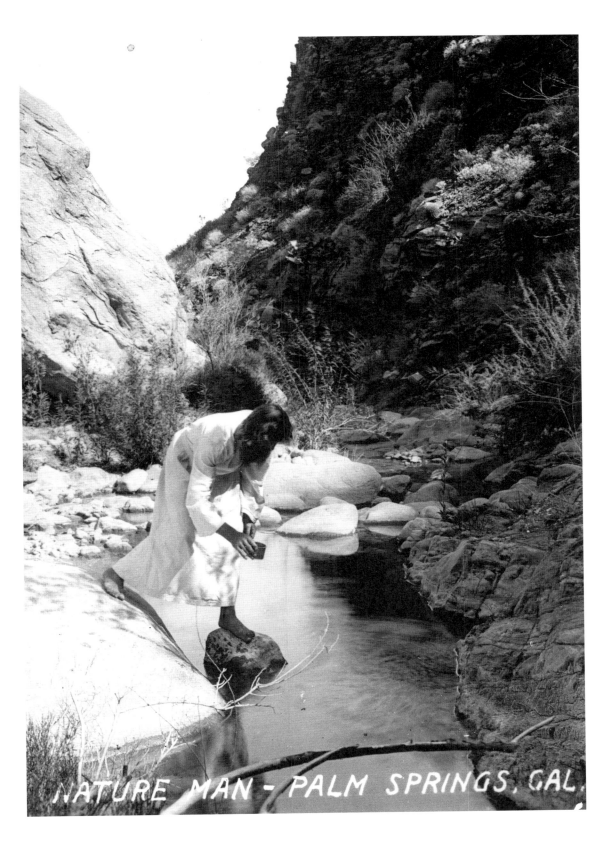

NATURE MAN - PALM SPRINGS, CAL.

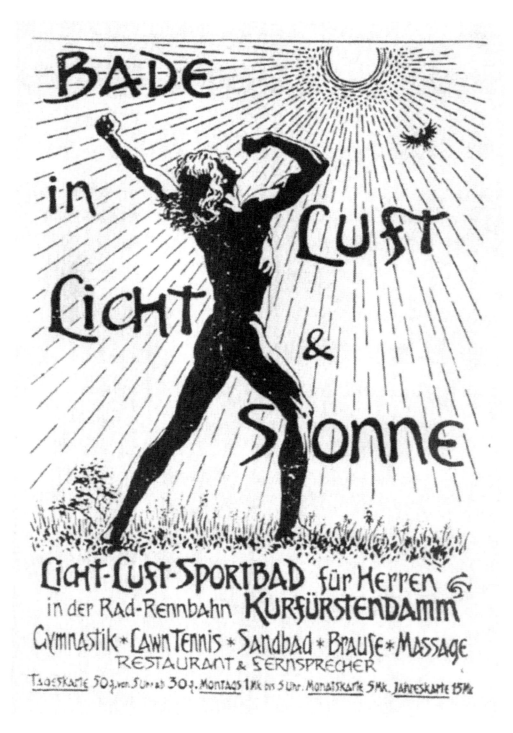

116   Advertisement for a new Light-Air-Sportbath for men in Berlin, reading
"Bathe in Air Light & Sun" by Fidus (Hugo Höppener), circa 1901.

ZURÜCK ZUR NATUR!

While Pester was unusual, he was not an anomaly. His lifestyle was rooted in the progressive movements that had spread across Europe and the United States in the nineteenth century. The particular philosophies and aims of these groups ranged widely, but most focused on one or a blend of health reform (diet, exercise, clothing, hygienic dwellings), political reform (anti-capitalist, anarchist, socialist, pacifist), and social reform (suffrage, child-labor, sexual mores). In the words of one historian, utopian-minded reformists of this era, intent on dismantling and re-forging all aspects of society, "swam in a sudden abundance of solutions."

In Pester's homeland, various reformist movements were known under the catch-all term *Lebensreform* (life reform). Its adherents, usually of the bourgeoisie, shared the belief that civilization itself required drastic rehabilitation. Their rallying cry was *Zurück zur Natur!* (Return to nature!)

"The iron cage weighed heaviest, and the fight against it was fiercest, in Germany," notes historian Martin Green. At the turn of the last century, the majority of Germans were modernizing alongside their teeming and increasingly polluted cities. They witnessed a parade of new inventions such as automobiles, radio, moving pictures, or the occasional phenomenon of a zeppelin drifting across the sky. Their nation was experiencing the most extreme pace of industrialization and urban growth in Europe. Centuries of tradition were broken as rural families moved to live near mines or manufacturing plants. Military spending nearly doubled and resources were stretched thin as the bulging colonial German empire raced to seize more territory around the world. By 1910, Germany contained as many large cities as the entirety of the rest of the continent combined.

HERMITS IN THE CANYONS

The fight against this 'iron cage' took several remarkable and reactionary forms, all striving to bend civilization back toward a more natural state. Some of Lebensreform's more ardent adherents were given the moniker *Naturemenschen* (nature people, or naturals). They lived simply and wore their hair long and clothes loose, leaving cities and societal pressures behind. A few wandered through Germany barefoot, preaching their dogma of a natural way of life. They were the eccentrics of their time, often mocked or derisively called '*Kohlrabi-Heiliger*' (cabbage saints) for their vegetarianism and evangelistic air.

Some, like Pester, left Europe behind. Others tried to form their own separate societies. Their efforts resembled the retreat to pursue cures at pastoral sanatoriums, except that the 'illness' was civilization itself. One Naturmensch, the pacifist and artist Karl Wilhelm Diefenbach, left Munich in 1886 with his family (including a son named Helios) to found a short-lived rural commune in an abandoned quarry. He then moved to Vienna, where his long beard and hair, bare feet, and rough-hewn cowl and tunic made him a spectacle—and a target of the police. In 1897 he founded a second, larger operation called Himmelhof on the city's outskirts. About two dozen like-minded men and women joined Diefenbach to live communally and follow his strict rules on free love, nude sun-bathing, and nature worship, until the venture went bankrupt two years later.

One of the residents at Himmelhof, the similarly clad artist and poet Gustav Gräser, took part in founding another, more durable living-experiment in the fishing village of Ascona, Switzerland. In 1900, Gräser and a small group of progressive Europeans gathered near the shore of Lake Maggiore to create their own "co-operative vegetarian colony." They named it 'Monte Verità' (Mountain of Truth). Another of its founders, the writer and feminist Ida Hofmann,

right — Round dance of the first vegetarians, Monte Verità, Ascona, Switzerland, circa 1910.

hoped it would provide an alternative to the "egoism, luxury, appearance, and lies" of modern life, not to mention of marriage: that "chain of intolerable lies." Monte Verità's reputation spread widely, and over the years it attracted a motley group of anarchists, dancers, long-hairs, proto-psychedelic artists, occultists, Tolstoyan ascetics, sandal-wearers, and healers. A large vegetable garden was tended, sans clothing, and a nature-cure sanatorium financed the operation. Some visitors stayed for years, living in loosely slatted 'light-and-air huts' or even caves. Others just passed through, perhaps meeting at dawn for a nude sun salute.

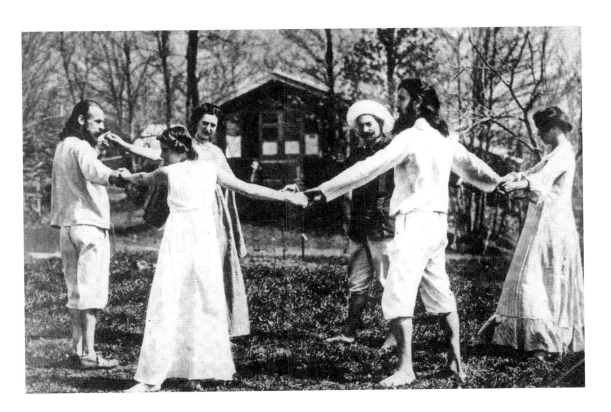

119

Monte Verità became known as a center for those seeking a new and freer lifestyle, attracting widely known personalities like Isadora Duncan, Carl Jung, Alexei Jawlensky, H.G. Wells, Rudolf Steiner, and Hermann Hesse. Less renowned but more central to our tale was the tenure of the blazing health reformer Arnold Ehret, who spread his gospel of fasting and raw food along the shore of the sparkling lake before eventually bringing it to Los Angeles circa 1920.

The tenets of Lebensreform, while always on the fringes of society, also manifested in highly organized, even institutionalized systems. In 1896, a group of teenaged boys studying shorthand in a Berlin suburb began organizing long nature hikes. These outings appeared to be a pleasant group exercise, but their immersion in nature expressed a heady sense of freedom and a critique of modern society. The participants, all boys at first, dressed eccentrically for their hikes, as gypsies or troubadours, in tattered capes, romantic collars and bright scarves, with hiking boots, walking sticks and backpacks. Drawing inspiration from Germany's pagan and Medieval past, the excursions were akin to walking backwards in time. By 1901 their growing movement was formalized and named *Wandervogel* (wandering bird), and eventually other boys started their own local chapters.

"Our people need whole men, not fragments such as notaries, party hacks, scholars, officials, and courtiers," claimed an article in *Wandervogel* magazine. As one member wrote, the movement created "an honest world, not the world of illusions that was called 'society.'" Another article underscored this credo:

"Through hiking, the city boy breaks the habit of perceiving every gust of wind, every rain shower, every wet boot as another nail in his coffin. Instead he... ventures out, laughing, into the wind and the rain. So go out into forest and field, German boys, and open your eyes to the life and

activity of nature. Long live hiking, which sharpens the senses and keeps the spirit pure and fresh!"

When their long rambles throughout Germany and Switzerland extended into overnight excursions, the Wandervogel would sleep in clubhouses they called 'nests' or 'anti-homes.' As night fell, the youths gathered around bonfires under open skies, sang traditional songs, strummed guitars and lutes, and told fanciful folktales. In some ways they resembled the outdoor scouting movements arising around the same time in the United States and England, except they were youth-led and scorned the adult world of obligatory etiquette and toil. There were no badges to win and no patriotism to pledge except to a fabled remnant of ancient Germania. Spending long periods in natural settings tapped into a deep thirst for freedom, fortitude, and authenticity. Within thirteen years of its founding, an estimated 50,000 Wandervogel members had joined from schools across the country, heeding the cry: "So go out into forest and field, German boys."

The yearning for a more natural state also manifested in 'physical culture,' an area of reformist thinking focused on making the healthy body stronger and more beautiful, and in turn, viewing such bodies as evidence of moral minds. For men, physical culture often manifested in sports and bodybuilding; for women, graceful exercises such as dance. All were considered most effective if pursued in the nude. The uncovered body signified an authentic, less artificial way of being. One German magazine of the era proclaimed: "Nudity equals truth."

Richard Ungewitter, one of nudism's earliest and most extreme proponents, agreed. As he sat naked at his polished wooden desk in Stuttgart, he wrote reams of overwrought prose promoting communal nudism, vegetarianism, and racial purity. Published in the first few years of the twentieth century, his books sold over

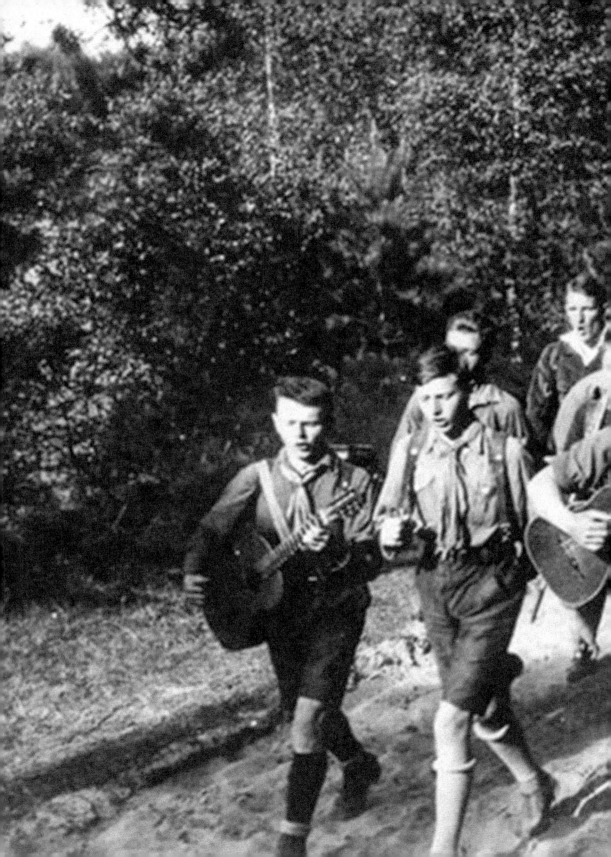

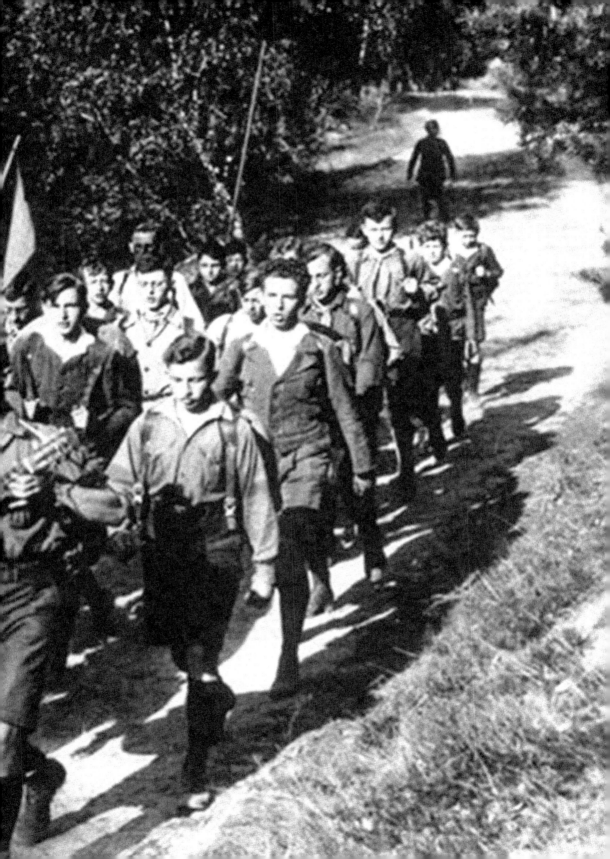

100,000 copies. To Ungewitter, nudity was a way to shed the forces of capitalism and socialism, exposing the pure, uncontaminated German spirit. The body was celebrated—but only certain types.

Several other popular nudism manifestos were published in Germany at the turn of the century and found a wide readership. Most advocates linked nude exercise to its practice in ancient Greece and, like the Wandervogel movement, viewed an embrace of nature as a means to reclaim an idealized past. Nudism was also considered a pathway to better health (many advocates cited tubercular statistics in their arguments) and a way of displaying the fruits of a good diet and active lifestyle—which in turn proved a superior and intelligent mind. The classical notion of *mens sana in corpore sano* (a healthy mind in a healthy body) was a touchstone.

Germany's first *Freilichtpark* (free-light park) for nudists opened near Hamburg in 1903. Similar parks and nudist clubs proliferated throughout the nation and were later founded in France and England. Nudity was institutionalized in open-air schools for ill or delicate children, while nude gymnastics classes were offered as a way of strengthening the body while exposing it to the healing properties of air and light. (Meanwhile on the sandy beaches of Los Angeles, men were arrested for sunbathing topless as late as 1929.)

After the First World War, the perception of the nude body shifted and intensified. As historian Paul Overy has noted, the bared, healthy body was now celebrated for its symbolic wholeness in opposition to the mutilation and decimation of millions of men in Europe's trenches. During the postwar years, images of nude bodies in natural landscapes formed an antipode to city life and the mechanical killing machines of war. In the 1919 German silent film *Nerven* (*Nerves*), for example, scenes depict anguished urban characters melodramatically wringing their hands and lamenting

previous page — A group of Wandervogel youth from Berlin on a long journey, circa 1930.

their misery. At the end of the story, two protagonists break free and ascend a sunny hillside to gaze upon the splendor of a craggy mountain range. They shed their clothes, embracing in loincloths. The woman nestles against the man as he raises his arms in a triumphant V toward the sun. The final intertitle reads, "Return to Nature!"

A few years later, Berliner Hans Surén published *Der Mensch und die Sonne (Man and Sunlight),* featuring photographs of deeply tanned nude men and women modeling and flexing in bright sunlight. The author himself was often featured in these images, his browned skin oiled as he struck muscular poses in a tiny loincloth. Surén's asexual paean to the nude body proved wildly popular; it was reprinted 61 times in its first year (1924) and translated into several languages.

By the end of the 1920s, the intensity of German allegiance to the sun and its impact on the body was recorded quite memorably by British poet and novelist Stephen Spender. Upon visiting Hamburg he wrote:

"The sun... was a primary social force in this Germany. Thousands of people went to the open-air swimming baths or lay down on the shores of the rivers and lakes, almost nude, and sometimes quite nude, and the boys who had turned the deepest mahogany walked amongst those people with paler skins, like kings among their courtiers. The sun healed their bodies of the years of war, and made them conscious of the quivering, fluttering life of blood and muscles covering their exhausted spirits like the pelt of an animal: and their minds were filled with an abstraction of the sun, a huge circle of fire, an intense whiteness blotting out the sharp outlines of all other forms of consciousness, burning out even the sense of time."

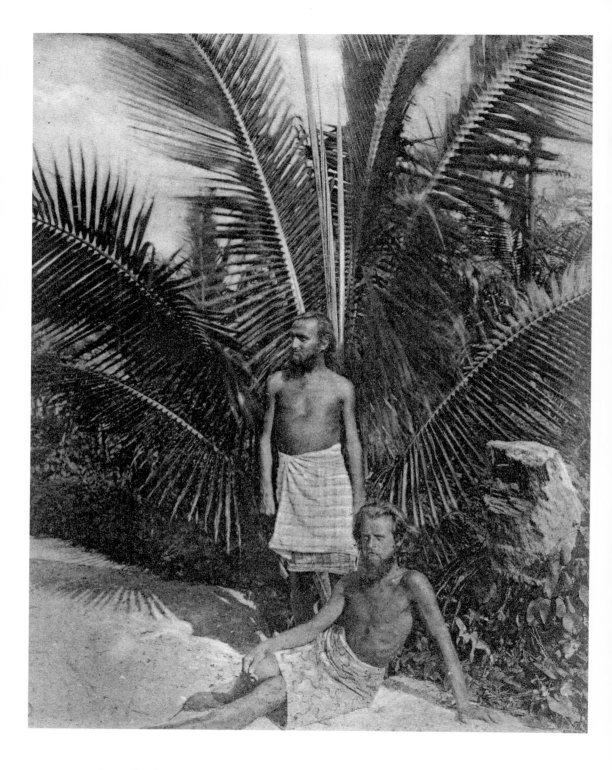

August Engelhardt under a palm tree with concert pianist Max Lützow at his feet, circa 1902. Lützow joined Engelhardt's nudist, coconut-centric community, *Sonnenorden* (Order of the Sun), and ultimately died there.

While the reform movements blazed especially bright in Germany, the sense that civilization had grown intractably corrupt was felt in other parts of Europe and the United States as well. This backlash might have seemed urgent and new, but it was not. The urge to return to nature is perpetual philosophical ballast against surges of industrialization. (Some historians have traced this impulse all the way back to ancient Rome.) The greater the surge, it seems, the stronger the backlash.

In the eighteenth century the influential Swiss philosopher Jean-Jacques Rousseau had advocated a more natural way of life, declaring: "Cities are the abyss of the human species." In Massachusetts in 1845, Henry David Thoreau famously retreated to pastoral life at Walden Pond, demoralized by the routine of industrialized modern life. "Men have become the tools of their tools," he lamented. "We need the tonic of wildness."

Civilization was not just a source of physical illness, to be treated with a change of climate or more sanitary housing, but a spiritual threat. Its benefits were vigorously questioned by a new generation of crusaders reacting to rapid changes, from urban density and the drudgery and alienation of modern labor, to the compression of time launched by speeding trains and telegraphs. The psychic malady of the era was often diagnosed as 'neurasthenia,' a vague condition characterized by lassitude, nervousness, and overstimulation. Civilization—metallic, hurried, roaring—was the catch-all disease. Nature was the antidote.

"Thousands of tired, nerve-shaken, over-civilized people are beginning to find out going to the mountains is going home," wrote famed naturalist John Muir in California. Neglecting a relationship to nature was seen as perilous to one's mental health. "Once let the human race be cut off from personal contact with the soil," warned an American physician in 1888, "once let the conventionalities and artificial restrictions of so-called civilization interfere with the healthful simplicity of nature, and decay is certain."

In 1889 in England, poet and socialist Edward Carpenter published his lecture "Civilisation: Its Cause and Its Cure," which enjoyed numerous reprintings (and drew such admirers as author and vegetarian Leo Tolstoy). Carpenter, a fan of Indian mysticism and openly homosexual, lived simply on a few rural acres where he grew his own food and made sandals for his friends. He disdained shoes as "leather coffins" and believed civilization was a dark period, a disease that humans had to pass through like a bout of sickness. Carpenter's book on civilization opens with a quote from a thinker he greatly revered, Walt Whitman:

"The friendly and flowing savage... who is he? Is he waiting for civilization or past it and mastering it?"

This was the question that absorbed Carpenter and many of his contemporaries who were trying to understand the disturbing state of artifice and corruption produced by progress. Was it progress? Or its opposite? And who, if the over-civilized European had failed, might offer a way out? Versions of Whitman's "friendly and flowing savage" were a common answer. It led to many a vexing scene.

In turn-of-the-century America, the wilderness, and a confident, harmonious relation to it, were seen as invigorating for the Caucasian body and mind, especially for a developing youth under threat of being weakened by urban life. The newly popular activities of camping and scouting offered an immersion in nature, and ample opportunities for 'playing Indian.' Girls learned how to sew and embroider indigenous-style ceremonial costumes, plaiting their hair into long braids and wearing beaded moccasins, while boys acquired outdoor survival skills. In the Connecticut woods in around 1902, a boys' scouting group called the 'Woodcraft Indians' formed a fictional tribe called 'The Sinaways.' They engaged in mimicry of Native American culture complete with teepees, feather headdresses, and a hodgepodge of manly outdoor rituals. (What sins were being brushed away by the borrowed play-acting of The Sinaways, we know not.)

"The Red Man is the apostle of outdoor life," declared Woodcraft's founder, Canadian author and naturalist Ernest Thompson Seton. During summer days the Woodcraft boys ran free in the forest and swam in the lake, as Seton witnessed their "arms white as milk" darken into the "brown sinewy arm of the Indian." In the evenings they gathered around camp-fires for their leader's tales of noble Indian glory, but, as Seton clarified, "with all that is bad and cruel left out." A few years later, Seton went on to co-found the North American Boy Scouts.[1]

Tales of North American indigenous tribes also captivated Europeans at the time, in particular Germans, who read the bestselling American Wild West adventure novels of Karl May faster than he could write them. (May remains the top-selling German author of all time.) May's romanticized stories told of the noble escapades of Winnetou, an Apache chief, and his best friend and blood brother Old Shatterhand, a German frontiersman.

William Pester likely read Karl May as a dreamy youth in Germany. When he settled in the Californian desert, Pester chose a lush canyon on the Cahuilla tribe's reservation. A census survey from 1920 lists him as the only foreigner among 20 members of the

1. During his time with the Woodcrafts, Ernest Thompson Seton wrote a letter to the editor of *The Journal of the Outdoor Life*, produced at Dr. Trudeau's sanatorium in Saranac Lake, applauding the doctor for his emphasis on the outdoor cure and suggesting he add some teepees for their picturesque effect. The letter was published on the journal's front page. However, Seton's views were not always celebrated. In 1915, five years after the North American Boy Scouts was founded, Seton resigned due to a widening ideological gap between its founders. During the First World War, Seton's embrace of Indian customs was perceived as unpatriotic and he, in turn, rejected the Boy Scout's shift toward increasingly militaristic activities.

HERMITS IN THE CANYONS

BOYS CAMPED AT WYNDYGOUL
"CAMP OF POCATOPOG TRIBE"

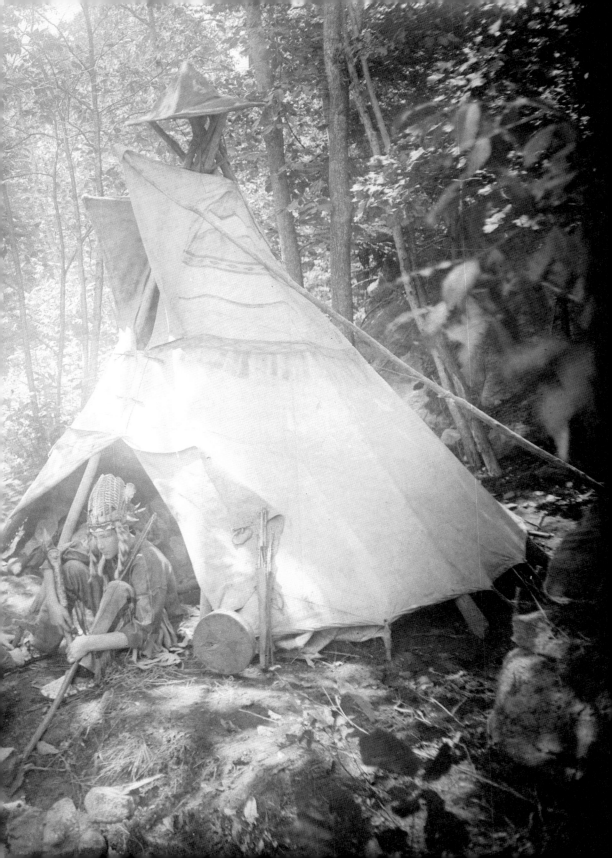

tribe living there. Debates persist about whether the Cahuilla embraced or just tolerated the foreigner in their midst. But it seems likely that Pester would have needed their help to learn how to survive.

A few years before Pester left Germany, his compatriot, August Engelhardt, departed for a tiny island in what was then known as German New Guinea (now part of Papua New Guinea). His intention was to leave civilization behind forever and establish a new, all-natural nudist society based on the consumption of two life sources: the sun and coconuts. His bizarre endeavor made international headlines. Over the years fifteen young German men, wanting to join his 'Order of the Sun,' followed him to renounce society and worship the orb of white fire in the South Seas. None lived long. Engelhardt himself perished there, emaciated but deeply tanned.

Meanwhile a baffling photograph from 1905 shows a group of unnamed, pale-chested men in Berlin lined up at a hospital during their "light-and-air bath." Most sport the closely cropped hair and coiffed mustaches of the era. But they are all barefoot and wearing only dried grass skirts resembling those of some tropical island culture. Playing Indian, even in the city, was apparently part of their health regimen.

previous page — Boys camped on Ernest Thompson Seton's estate in Connecticut, acting as the "Pocatopog" tribe, circa 1908.

Returning to nature had different ramifications for women. Carrica Le Favre, the spirited founder of vegetarian societies in New York and Boston, published her instructive guide for women, *Mother's Help and Child's Friend*, in 1890. Quite progressive—if not eccentric for its time—the book advocated a strict meat-free diet of milk and vegetables for children, and for open windows and fresh air in the nursery. But above all it underlined the moral and patriotic imperative of child-rearing. She decried women who tried to exert influence in the political arena, explaining that they "have an incomparably greater scepter in the pliable young heart and brain at home in the cradle."

While there was a celebrated strength and nobility attained by men returning to a more 'natural' masculinity, the notion of natural femininity was often circumscribed by its most biological role: motherhood. The spheres of the home, childcare, and elementary education offered the least threatening testing ground for reform. To push too far at these parameters was to threaten the notion of womanhood itself. Hence the claim by an American biologist in 1914 that suffragists were not women at all, but "mistakes of Nature."

Still, women found ways to return to nature, warily eyeing the line between radical and demure. In 1905 Dr. Bess Mensendieck, an American-born physician based in Vienna, published *Korperkultur der Frau* (*Body Culture of Women*), a guide to her exercise regimen of 53 'natural' movements. Full of photographs of impassive nude women and girls performing the exercises, her system proved very popular, and she established a wide network of girls' movement schools across Central and Northern Europe. The exercises aimed to strengthen the female body and make it nimbler, but they were often quotidian and domestically oriented. Movements associated with ironing clothes, reading a

133

book, carrying a tray, or lifting a baby were given the gravitas of ballet.

Despite the popularity of Mensendieck's theories, most nudist advocates were men, and their thoughts about female nudity and bodily health were bound by procreational goals. With his usual shrill dogmatism, the naked German scribe Richard Ungewitter wrote that nudism among women would serve to re-focus their attention on the strength and beauty of their bodies to the benefit of their husbands and future children.

While women faced exclusion from some of the reforms their brethren enjoyed, the realms of natu-ropathic and hydropathic medicine, in particular, offered rare entry. Women were accepted as doctors and healers long before traditional medical schools admitted them. Mid-nineteenth-century nature-cure advocates were some of the first to promote simple, loose clothing for women, pointing out the hazards of tight lacing and hauling around pounds of petticoats and bustles.[2] For example, Dr. Kellogg, at his Battle Creek Sanitarium, vehemently rejected the notion that women were inherently weaker or prone to illness, and prescribed them the same regimen of diet, fasting, and exercise that men received. Historian Patricia A. Cunningham notes: "While many of [the health-reform doctors] sought good health for women to improve their existence in the domestic sphere, others sought good health for women so they could take their places in society—that is, in the public sphere."

A few years after the founding of the all-male Wandervogel movement, a group of bourgeois German women ventured out of their homes, shedding rigid hats, pristine gloves, and starched, high-necked garments. They donned more relaxed dress and sometimes added soft hats with jaunty feathers. With backpacks and walking sticks they, too, set off into the countryside for their own version of Wandervogel,

right — Pupils exercising at the Mensendieck School in Oslo, Norway, in the 1950s.

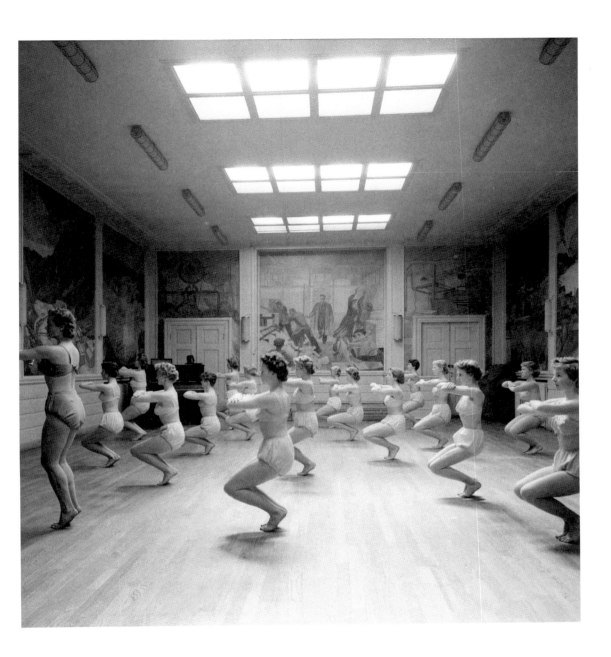

2. While the new flowing outfits were certainly more 'natural' than what had come before, they were curiously marketed with inverse terms, such as 'business' or 'science'. Loose dresses over leggings or billowing pants were named "Women's Practical Business Costumes" at the Battle Creek Sanitarium (where they were sold to all incoming patients). Ardent American dress reformer Mary Tillotson, who claimed to have healed her dyspepsia by shortening her dress hem by 12 inches, deemed her design a "Science Costume."

135

roaming freely from the confines of their lives. The *Bund der Wanderschwestern* (League of Wandering Sisters) was formed after Marie Luise Becker, a reformist and widow of a Wandervogel enthusiast, circulated a pamphlet articulating the need for a similar autonomous women's group:

"For much too long the limited focus on school, class and parenthood hindered the development of our girls... For the good of the German people we want to bring up mothers who are at home in the forests, meadows and pastures, who have learnt to listen to nature, have strengthened their health with amiable walking and have developed an eye for all things mighty and beautiful."

Her call attracted many hundreds of women. But even with its emphasis on "bringing up mothers," it was controversial. Wanderlust was considered inappropriate for unsupervised young women; a desire for wildness (or wilderness) suggested loose morals and the threat of an earthy sensuality. As it turned out, the women wanderers received the most criticism not from their parents or conservative elders, but from the male members of the Wandervogel, who saw the movement as a specifically masculine connection to nature.[3] When the young men returned from fighting in the First World War, they were dismayed to find their pastoral refuge 'feminized' by the swelling numbers of women who had taken on leadership roles. They immediately attempted to expel them.

REFORM CORRUPTED

By the 1930s in Germany, aspects of Lebensreform were swept into the rising tide of fascism. One example of this swift undertow is seen in the path of Leni Riefenstahl's film career. She was an actress and dancer before she became the Third Reich's favored filmmaker. In 1925 she danced in the silent film *Wege zu Kraft und Schönheit* (*Paths to Strength and Beauty*), an emblematic celebration of the physical culture and back-to-nature movements. Scenes depict urban laborers bent over sewing machines or paperwork, and the X-ray of a twisted, beleaguered spine. But outdoor movement, sport, and dance offer liberation, as shown in joyous scenes of lithe women and men in loincloths demonstrating their agility. (One sequence pays tribute to the Mensendieck method.) An ending shot shows the chilling vision of marching soldiers, but the intertitle states, "Today it is not military drills, but sports that are the source of a nation's strength." Just ten years later, in 1935, Riefenstahl released her propaganda film *Triumph of the Will*, filled with scenes of military drills. The Aryan body, strengthened by sunshine and movement, hardened by hiking and fresh air, was molded into a patriotic device, ready for war or childbirth.

The Third Reich expunged certain tenets of the Lebensreform movements, razing communes and criminalizing pacifism, while co-opting those that served its aims. Opponents who could escape the fascist tide, fled. Flowing hair on men, not to mention free thinking, was decidedly out of favor. When the Nazi Party seized power in 1933, Wandervogel was

---

3. Not only were female Wandervogel groups mocked, satirized, and shown hostility by some of the men, but when a history of the movement was being written in the 1960s, the author, Werner Kindt, claimed to have "lost" the many letters and documentation sent to him by female members. When historian Marion E. P. de Ras and other scholars discovered the material 20 years later, it was unopened.

dismantled in order to regroup young people under the banner of Hitler Youth. The tradition of organized hiking and folk nostalgia morphed into military camps and marching. Likewise, the widespread nudism movement was briefly outlawed, purged of dissidents, then reconsolidated under state control. Hans Surén's nudist book, *Man and Sunlight,* was reprinted numerous times throughout the 1930s, and its embedded racism became more explicit after Surén joined the Nazi Party. In its later editions, subtitled *The Aryan-Olympian Spirit,* the racial hygiene rhetoric of Hitler and Goebbels flanked Surén's images of muscular, nude Aryan men. As historian Christian Adam notes, such images "didn't just hold the promise of freedom. They also held thoughts of breeding—the body as a breeding tool that must be properly trained and fed like a race horse." Even the diets favored by many in the Lebensreform movement were carried forward: Hitler himself publicly abstained from tobacco and alcohol and was an occasional, but vocal, vegetarian and briefly a raw food advocate. By law during his regime, bakeries were encouraged to produce wholegrain bread, and soybeans, celebrated as an excellent source of strengthening protein, were bizarrely renamed 'Nazi beans.'

right — Demonstration of exercises from Hans Surén's *Atemgymnastik,* 1929.

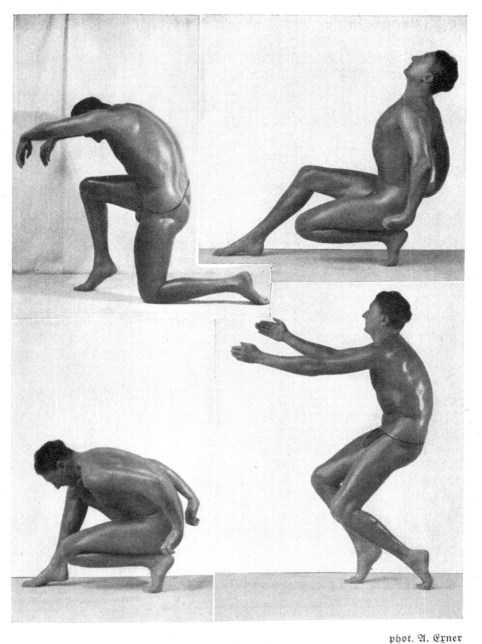

phot. A. Exner

Abb. 84—87
Surén-Körperschule. Einfache Atemflußübung von links oben nach rechts unten
= wechselnde Aus- und Einatmung

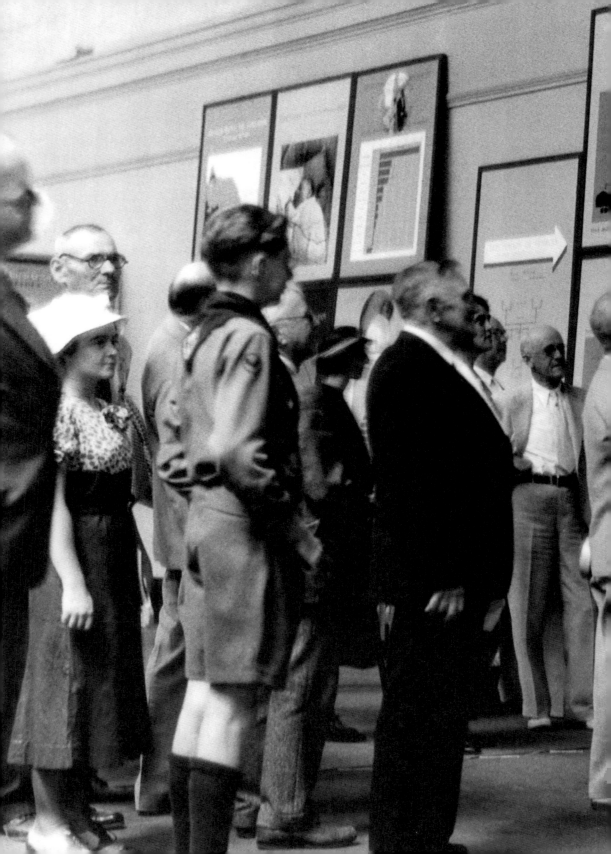

I t's tempting to view the different strands of the reformist movements in black and white. In Germany, the seemingly benign pursuits of nude gymnastics, organized hiking, and resurrecting old folk songs torqued down a sinister path to war and depravity. Exported elsewhere, they led to very different outcomes and many positive social advances. But the movement had stealthily carried a virus for decades. Since the late nineteenth century many progressives in the United States and Europe, from pacifists to birth control advocates, had embraced the new 'science' of eugenics, the process of selective breeding and sterilization. It was viewed as a rational, benevolent way to engineer a utopian society of the fittest. Also called 'racial hygiene,' or 'race betterment,' eugenics was considered one of many efforts, like sleeping with the windows open, that would forge a healthier population.

I Wish They All Could be California Girls

In California the superior climate and agriculture aroused not only wild claims about optimum health, but also declarations about its potential to advance the human body, and thus, the species. As Walt Whitman predicted about the American West in 1858:

"Here the air is dry and antiseptic—everything grows to a size, strength, and expanse, unknown in the Northern and Eastern States. Nature is on a large scale; and here, in time to come, will be found a wonderful race of men."

Fueled by anxiety over extensive immigration, the state participated in the popular pseudo-scientific practice of measuring the physical and 'moral' strengths among different types of people to determine ideal genetic outcomes. (Nationwide, those doing the measuring were primarily of Anglo-Saxon or Nordic stock; their race always placed highest.) One proponent of this pursuit was David Starr Jordan, respected scientist and first president of northern California's Stanford University, who declared that California-born college-aged women were taller, broader, stronger, and had more lung capacity than women of the same age in Massachusetts. Such pronouncements were commonplace. In 1929, articles in Los Angeles newspapers claimed that California's athletes were becoming the nation's greatest due to fresh vitamin-rich fruits and having more "solidified sunshine" in their hearts and muscles. Bodily strength and health could reach new heights in the Golden State, some asserted, and a superior species—sun-filled, vital, and longer-living—would eclipse the old.

But only if this promising gene pool was limited. (Interracial marriage between certain groups had been outlawed in the state in 1850.) California was third in the nation to legalize forced sterilizations, in 1909, and over the years it outpaced other states (per capita) for the quantity of procedures. The sterilizations ostensibly targeted criminals and the mentally ill, but were disproportionately practiced on people of non-European descent. This American project was of great interest to the nascent Nazi regime in the 1920s.[1] However once the number of coercive sterilizations in Germany was made public, operating at a pace up to twenty times more aggressive than that of the United States, its popularity elsewhere withered overnight.

continued from overleaf — **Display of the exhibit "Eugenics in New Germany" at the American Public Health Association meeting in Pasadena, California, 1934.**

1. In as late as 1935 a eugenics think tank based in Long Island sent a genetic chart from California for presentation at a eugenics conference in Germany. It showed an 'unfit' family tree and the sterilization that would halt its propagation.

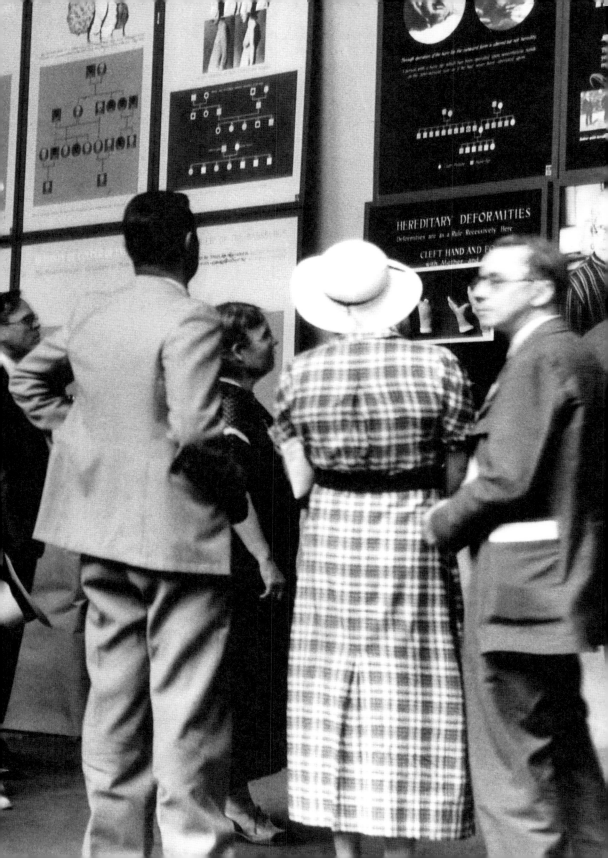

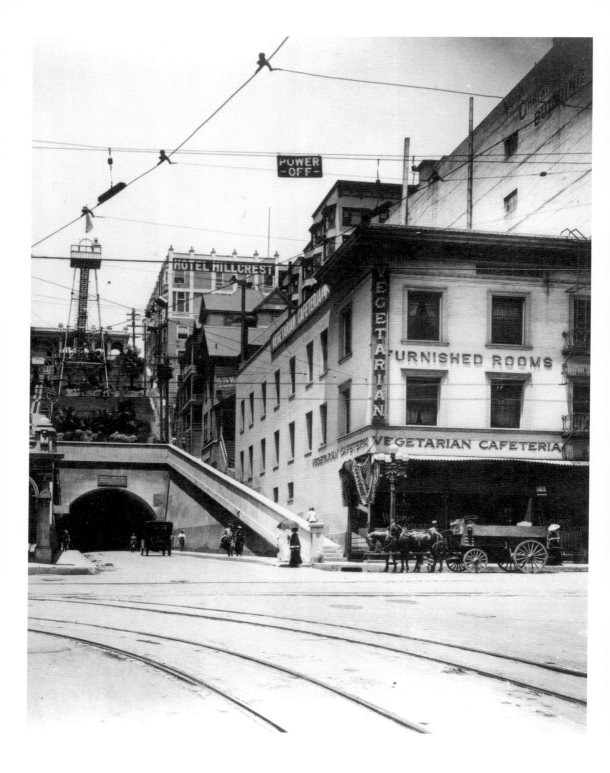

144   Vegetarian Cafeteria on the corner of 3rd & Hill streets, by Angels Flight, Downtown
Los Angeles, California.

THERE IS DEATH IN THE POT

"Los Angeles! Where religion turns into thousands of obscure cults; whereby street dress men and women merge into a common sex; and where the fine art of eating becomes a pseudo scientific search for a lost vitality hidden in the juice of a raw carrot."
– Works Progress Administration (WPA) government report, 1930s

On a typical morning around 1920, Vera Richter could be found scooping ground carob into a pile of chopped dates and raisins, then forming the sticky brown mixture into a loaf and setting it on a windowsill to 'bake' for several hours in the California sun. When it was ready, she sliced it up to serve at the Raw Food Dining Room, a restaurant in Downtown Los Angeles she ran with her husband John, a kindly-looking man with short gray hair and round spectacles. The walls of their eclectic restaurant were decorated with a photograph of President Woodrow Wilson on one side and of Eugene Debs, leader of the Socialist Party of America, on the other. Above Debs's portrait was a copy of the recently adopted Soviet constitution. Languid Hawaiian music spun on the phonograph while diners sipped cups of coconut-lemon or flaxseed juice and tucked into bowls of uncooked soups, plates of vegetable and flower salads, or Vera's sun-cooked 'unfired' pies. Also on display were the pro-Bolshevik leaflet *The Truth about Russia* and the restaurant's credo: "Raw food, plus sunshine, air and exercise promotes physical, moral, mental and spiritual health."

Founded in 1917, the Richters' restaurant was the city's and the country's first raw vegetarian dining establishment—and possibly the world's. It was a fitting location; the small agricultural city of Los Angeles had been host to vegetarian restaurants since the turn of the century. And for 30 years before that, the region claimed at least two short-lived religious vegetarian sects, plus sanatoriums and health resorts that served and sold vegetarian products, reaping the benefits of abundant fresh produce.

In 1880 the *Baltimore Sun* described Los Angeles as a haven for vegetarians, where the sunny winter months offered so much more than the limited, snowbound repetition of "stewed cabbage, boiled rice, and dried apples":

"Los Angeles, California, is one of the few spots on the globe where the strict vegetarian would be able to find free pasturage all the year... You can always find fresh fruit in Los Angeles, and it may be plucked from the tree or vine the whole year round. The lemon and the lime are in bearing there the livelong year, and the orange reigns from Christmas to July; apples and pears are on the trees from July until November, and then may be kept till Spring; peaches come in as early as June 15th, and do not disappear until Christmas; grapes are in season five months, and so also are plums and prunes; the guava ripens nearly all the year; the berry season begins in May and lasts through September."

The region's reputation as a vegetarian sanctuary apparently spread very far. In 1883, a "curious feature of immigration" was noted by the author of the rapturous guidebook *Prosperous California: A Land of Money, Progress and Content.* A German "society of vegetarians, who believe that none but the vegetable should be eaten by the human race" was making plans to immigrate to the state. They had already tried and failed to establish roots in Honduras and Paraguay, and now selected the more welcoming climate of Los Angeles County. The author (whose name has been lost to history) added that the group's "leading spirits look forward to establishing a very large and flourishing colony of vegetarians in California in the near future." The fate of this particular group is unknown, but a flourishing colony, of a sort, was indeed established.

The state's long-standing renown, and the many invalids who flocked there for a cure, meant that restaurants like the Richters' had a built-in clientele, a group ready to break with convention and plunge into new territory for the sake of health—physical and spiritual. The region's horticultural riches were also a goldmine for the health entrepreneurs, from business-men to half-baked prophets, that Los Angeles raked in. A few of these players were homegrown; others had imported their fervor for health and diet from the Midwest or East Coast. But an outsized number drew directly from Germany, land of Lebensreform and nature-cure pioneers.

In the 1910s a black truck with wood-spoked wheels roamed the streets of Los Angeles selling dried fruits and nuts. The words "Carque's Pure Foods" were emblazoned on the side of this so-called 'health wagon.' As he drove along the partially paved streets, expat Otto Carque, a compact man with a thick moustache, might have shouted slogans from the window: "Get nature's foods! Pure fruits and nuts! All natural! Don't poison your body!" Carque had a German accent and a theatrical flair; he always carried around a black leather doctor's bag filled with samples of dried fruits and nuts along with his self-published health pamphlets. A friend referred to this bag as a symbol of the future doctor who would treat ailments with food, not drugs.

Carque had arrived in Los Angeles in 1905 and, enamored with the sweet musk of local Black Mission figs, saw an opportunity. He had the keen foresight to trademark the phrase "Natural Foods of California," and eventually traded in his health wagon for several health food stores in the 1920s. Local olives, juices, nut butters, freshly milled flours, whole grains, and dried fruits lined the shelves of his popular shops. His health philosophy was distilled into books as well as numerous articles for a wide range of magazines. (These magazines' titles offer a fitting snapshot of the varied, sometimes overlapping strands of the era's progressivism: Carque wrote and advertised in *The Vegetarian Magazine*, Bernarr Macfadden's *Physical Culture*, the *Journal of Eugenics*, *The American Theosophist*, and *The Indian's Friend*, a pro-Native magazine edited and published by concerned women in northeastern America.) Carque strongly promoted fresh air, hiking, and sunshine, and claimed to have invented the fruit-nut bar, or "Carque's California Fruit Bar," which provided "muscular energy and endurance for the traveler; long distance walker; and mountain climber." It may have been the first energy bar, although claims for that distinction are many.

Carque was continuing a long tradition of health evangelism wed to new products that are still with us today. In around 1829, a Presbyterian minister in Pennsylvania named Sylvester Graham invented the graham cracker, a whole-wheat cracker he believed would suppress sexual appetites. Besides its lust-dampening properties, Graham and his followers, the Grahamites, believed the crackers were a morally and physically healthier alternative to store-bought bread made with mechanically processed superfine flour and other dubious additives, which broke, as he fiercely argued, the "laws of the Creator."

A few decades later, at a small water-cure sanatorium in Western New York, Dr. James Caleb Jackson ushered the graham cracker into its next influential arena. An abolitionist and farmer-turned-physician, Jackson undertook to double-bake pieces of wet graham crackers, causing them to become more brittle. The result was a crispy, shard-like substance he called "granula." The cereal was tooth-breakingly hard when dry, so Jackson soaked the flakes in milk. After centuries of warm, cooked grains for breakfast, this was the first cold cereal.

One visitor to Jackson's sanatorium in around 1878 was Dr. John Kellogg, who would soon open the Sanitas Food Company at his vegetarian sanatorium in Battle Creek, Michigan. (A branch of Sanitas opened in Southern California in 1905.) After tasting Jackson's granula he developed his own version. Later on, Kellogg and his brother experimented with toasted, flattened flakes of dough, making the popular cereal that became known as corn flakes and launching the now-global Kellogg cereal empire. Kellogg's competitors took note, and several varieties of cold cereal flooded the market, giving way to what came to be called the great 'cereal boom' at the turn of the twentieth century.

Around the same time, in Switzerland, a young, bespectacled doctor named Maximilian Bircher-Benner was elevating mush with a dose of health-giving raw fruit. He believed raw food contained greater solar energy, a force lost through the process of cooking, and non-existent in animal flesh. Bircher-Benner sought a simple, cure-all dish that could easily deliver the benefits of what he deemed "sunlight food." Combining grated apple, lemon juice, sweetened condensed milk, nuts, and raw oats soaked in water, he developed his *Apfeldiätspeise* (apple dietary dish) in around 1900, prescribing it as a pre-meal starter or supper substitute. Eventually, the six-syllable meal acquired the nickname '*Müesli*', which means 'little mush.'

Back in Southern California, one of Carque's compatriots, a German emigrant named Hermann Sexauer, opened the first health food store in Santa Barbara, a small oceanside city north of Los Angeles. In Germany, Sexauer had been a member of both the German Vegetarian Society and the Wandervogel movement, but he left "to get away from the narrow-minded bour-geois at home, and to escape the stupidity and stifling influence of bureaucracy." He brought his vegetarian, pacifist, and anarchist views to the fertile ground of California around 1910. After years spent foraging fruits and olives on his bicycle and raising a family of four with his German botanist wife, he opened Sex-auer's Natural Foods in 1934. It was a gathering spot for like-minded health enthusiasts, offering an array of fresh produce, drugless healing tonics, and an impres-sive selection of European and American books on natural health, including those written by his allies in Los Angeles, the socialist raw-foodists John and Vera Richter.

Naturopathic medicine had been established in Southern California by way of the German couple Drs. Carl and Ellen Schultz. They founded the state's first naturopathic association in 1903 and fought doggedly to establish state legalization, which they won in 1909. The Schultzes ran the Naturopathic Institute and San-itarium in Downtown Los Angeles.

The Richters' restaurant was turning a profit and soon they were able to expand their operation, open-ing two raw-food restaurants Downtown. They named them the Eutropheon Live Food Cafeterias, borrowing the word from the ancient Greek *eutrophia*, meaning 'sound nutrition.' John offered free weekly lectures on the benefits of 'live' foods, while Vera labored on a volume of recipes and advice for natural living called *Mrs. Richter's Cook-less Book*. Her author photo shows a radiant, wholesome face, her dark hair cut into a chic bob. Published in 1924, it's thought to be the world's first raw vegan cookbook.

Years before he came to California John Richter had discovered the vegetarian, drugless system taught by Dr. Kellogg. He was an instant convert. It was already assumed that Richter would be a doctor, just like his German émigré father in Fargo, North Dakota, who owned a drug store where John learned how to compound prescriptions. But when John went to Chicago his interests diverged; he studied Kellogg's Battle Creek diet regimen and a Swedish system of movement exercises. When he returned home with a diploma in hand, his father immediately called him a quack. Then he asked permission to treat the patients his father had deemed incurable. As Richter recounts, nature-cure miracles ensued and his father promised to never call him a quack again.

Richter practiced naturopathic medicine and followed a vegetarian diet in the Midwest for about fifteen years but as he later recounted, "I was constantly harassed by a 'gone' feeling, lack of power to rebuild myself, in short, general lack of energy." In 1911 he learned of Benedict Lust, a German immigrant, publisher, and founder of America's first school of naturopathy.[4] Lust advocated a diet of uncooked, 'live foods.' As Richter recounted in his book *Nature, The Healer*:

"in a naturopathic magazine which had come to my hands, there was an article describing how a certain Dr. Lust had been invited... to partake of an uncooked food dinner. It told of the many different varieties of food that were served, of how delicious they were. It said something, too, about raw pie. I thought, 'How curious, unbaked pie!'"

Intrigued, Richter tried the diet for a few weeks and claimed to feel "reborn." "What a mental relief and assurance to know that I was getting better at last!" Galvanized by his new lifestyle he eventually headed to Los Angeles to open a raw-food restaurant and spread his discovery.

4. The school was founded in New York in 1901. Benedict Lust was arrested over a dozen times in the United States for practicing medicine without a license. He and his wife Luisa, also a naturopathic doctor, ran a water-cure sanatorium called Yungborn, in New Jersey, and both remain revered pioneers of present-day naturopaths.

HERMITS IN THE CANYONS

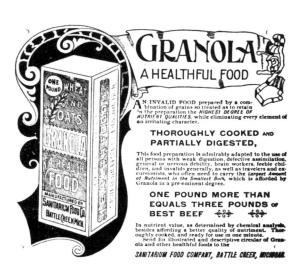
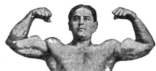
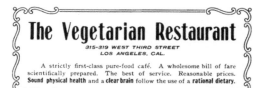
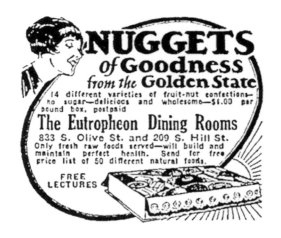
top left — Advertisement for Granola, circa 1893. bottom left — Advertisement for the Nature Cure Supply Centre, run by Benedict Lust. right — Advertisements for the Eutropheon and The Vegetarian restaurants.

It's unknown whether Vera, who was born in Pennsylvania, had come to a natural lifestyle on her own or after meeting John. But her enthusiasm was equally strong. One avid patron of the Eutropheon was Dr. Philip Lovell. As he had done with Rudolph Schindler, he invited Vera to be a guest writer for his column in the *Los Angeles Times*. Her dedication to raw foods, and her disdain of heated 'dead food,' was vehemently expressed:

"Can you visualize a master of wisdom bending over a cookstove, flavoring this, stirring that, making himself trouble, and raising much dust, and to what end? There is death in the pot. In a daily newspaper appeared a recipe for fried peaches. What a crime. A peach, beautiful and perfect in itself, with its organic qualities for man's refreshment, must be submitted to the destroying fire in order to gratify a perverted taste."

Heat and processing was believed to 'kill' the natural vitality of produce. "Under the process of cooking," she asserted, "the vitamins, so necessary to vigorous health, take wings and flee." Raw foods were seen as 'live' and full of life-giving energy—hence the name of the Eutropheon Live Food Cafeterias, and its slogan: "Live Food, Live People."

Mrs. Richter also had specific advice for women, calling on them to go further than casting off corsets and hoop skirts, and to discard "such unnecessary evils as furs, high-heeled shoes, face powders, rouge, etc." She advised natural beauty treatments such as using crushed raspberries or beet juice as rouge, eating raw carrots for glowing skin, and powdering the face with a porous bag of rolled oats. Her recommendations for women's health and happiness were to follow only the essential doctors of nature: Doctors Air, Light, Water, Fruit, Vegetable, Exercise, Recreation, and Sleep.

HERMITS IN THE CANYONS

This spirited scene was aided in its evangelism by the arrival of a wiry, charismatic German reformist with piercing eyes, shoulder-length hair, and a voluminous beard named Arnold Ehret. By 1920, Ehret was one of the city's legion of natural-healing advocates who lectured at the handful of vegetarian restaurants and health centers. In an article about an upcoming lecture of his at the Vital Food Dining Garden for members of the Longer Life League, it was expected that he'd be greeted with a rousing cheer of "Raw! Raw! Raw! Slaw! Slaw! Slaw!" before the group dug into alfalfa sprouts, salad, and, yes, more unfired pie.

Ehret's popularity was likely due to his direct link to European methods. He was touted as a "Swiss diet expert" and had roamed Europe experimenting with various nature cures, including a tenure at the lakeside bohemian colony of Monte Verità in Switzerland. Water and sun cures had his stamp of approval, but his favored method was a primarily raw diet and regular fasting. He found a small following in Los Angeles, regularly advertising his books, pamphlets, and lectures in the local newspaper and hawking his ability to "solve the FOOD and HEALTH problems."

Ehret referred to air as "sun-power" and fruit as "sun-food." He also claimed there was scientific proof that all sustenance the human body required could be found in apples, bananas, and coconuts.[5] Like many charismatic healers of the time, Ehret also manufactured and sold a cure-all natural remedy. His was called 'Innerclean,' an herbal laxative made from the yellow-flowered senna plant, and sold via post or at the small constellation of health-food stores and restaurants, including the Eutropheon. His advertisements became increasingly messianic, proclaiming he was the "GREATEST HEALER OF OUR TIMES," signed by twenty followers who argued, "HE IS THE TRUTH AND HAS THE TRUTH AND WE WITH HIM." Thus, the health-religion of 'Ehretism' was born. However, in

1922, after delivering a free and undoubtedly impassioned lecture Downtown, Ehret slipped on a puddle of automobile oil, struck his head on a curb, and died at the age of 56. As a tribute to his devotion to nature, his ashes are interred in an acorn-shaped urn.

Despite the death of its leader, Ehretism enjoyed a long afterlife. His local publishers and clients, the Hirsch brothers, held onto their faith, and their copyright of his books. They opened an Ehretist vegetarian retreat in 1927 called Highland Springs Health Resort in Beaumont, east of Los Angeles. The Hirsches also held 'Ehret demonstration dinners' into the 1930s and kept his books in circulation. Nearly a century later the books are still in print, and 'Arnold Ehret's Innerclean' is still sold.

The Richters, Carque, Sexauer, and Ehret were only a handful of the players who shaped the growing health scene in Southern California. The waves of influence were many, including a few vegetarian mystics from India who had enthralled large audiences since the turn of the century. Some health entrepreneurs gained celebrity, others invented products you can still find on the shelves of health-food stores. (The wordy proselytizing of these early zealots lives on in the labels of products like Dr. Bronner's soap and Dr. Bragg's apple cider vinegar.) The number of health entrepreneurs would only grow in the following decades, immeasurably aided by the new medium of moving pictures, which placed a premium on actors of astounding beauty and vigor whose larger-than-life faces and bodies flickered on screens in dark theaters. The alliance between movie stars and diet and exercise fanatics was inevitable—and enduring.

5. This particular strain of dietary thought, an ersatz tendril from Darwin's link between man and ape, was popular among Central Europe's more radical dietary connoisseurs. Recall August Engelhardt, who left Germany to subsist entirely on coconuts on a tropical island. If it served our jungle-dwelling primate forebears, the thinking went, it should serve humankind. Engelhardt's crusade was greatly admired by Ehret, who wrote reverently of him and considered joining him on his island. The two zealots shared a publisher for their fiery books: Benedict Lust.

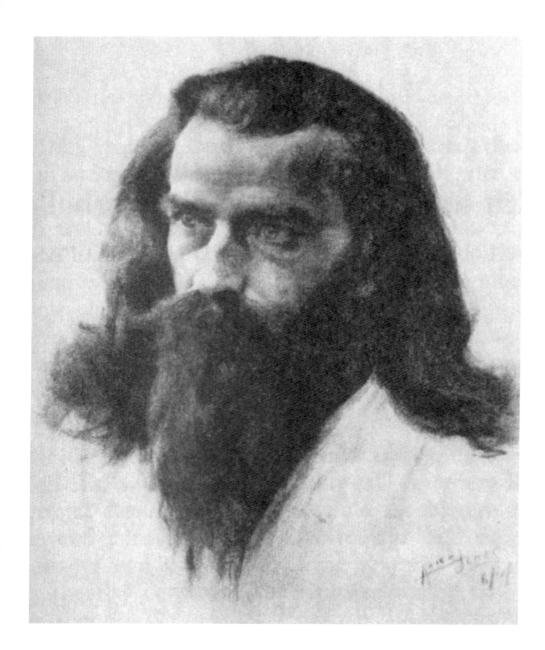

156   Portrait of Arnold Ehret.

The stage was set for a constant flow of strange diets and exercise regimens, all collected under a vague cloud of spiritual or utopian aspirations. One notorious health guru and organic restaurant owner in the 1970s changed his name to Father Yod, donned a long white beard, and famously started a free-love cult in an old Hollywood mansion.[6] His restaurant, The Source, served as a brief punchline about Los Angeles health food in the 1977 film *Annie Hall*, when a bewildered, consummate New Yorker visits and resignedly orders "alfalfa sprouts and a plate of mashed yeast."

6. Father Yod led a group of up to 200 white-clad vegetarian meditators called the Source Family. By odd coincidence the brick mansion they crowded into was originally built for the newspaper publisher Harry Chandler, an early naturopathic patient of Dr. Philip Lovell.

HERMITS IN THE CANYONS

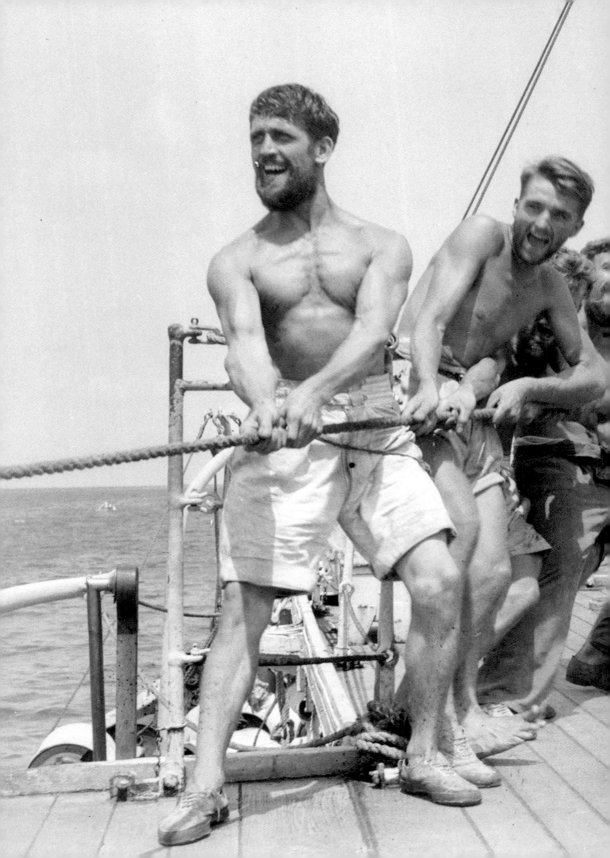

F or much of modern history, men in Europe were clean shaven. The regularly groomed bare face signaled enlightenment and a genteel respectability. Beards, in contrast, were viewed as waste matter, a mess that should be cleaned. If one chose to wade against this current by growing a beard, it was usually to express a radical break from social norms.

This all changed in 1850 in England, when beards became à la mode. Some have cited the Crimean War as the reason, noting the abundant beards soldiers grew to warm themselves during the fatally harsh winters on the front. This was influential but the causes were more complex. As historian Christopher Oldstone-Moore points out, the failure of social revolutions and political movements, such as Chartism (a parliamentary reform movement) in Britain also led to the shift. Once the culture-destabilizing aims of bearded renegades were no longer a threat, the style could be safely co-opted by the mainstream.

The full beard shed its extremist symbolism, instead signifying heroic masculinity available to men of all social classes. A flurry of pro-beard manifestos was published in the exclamatory prose of the era, such as: *The Beard! Why do We Cut it Off? An Analysis of the Controversy Concerning It, and An Outline of its History*; *Is Shaving Injurious to the Health? A Plea for the Beard*; and simply *Why Shave?* As labor moved indoors during the Industrial Age, men sought to re-assert their ruggedness; beards were popularized alongside atavistic bouts of hiking and hunting. As Oldstone-Moore notes, "true manhood was forged in the perils of rough nature: it was only appropriate that such men looked like men as nature made them." But pursuing nature was framed in the highest rational terms: "We live in an age both of progress and restoration," one essayist wrote in 1867, calling for the "restoration of the facial appendage to that part of the body where nature originally, and as we believe most kindly, implanted it. "Beards were also believed to possess health benefits, a theory that many doctors affirmed. In 1861 an army surgeon writing in *The Edinburgh Review* noted that clean-shaven military recruits suffered more bronchial infections than those "whose upper lips were plentifully clothed with hair." In a complete reverse of its former role, beards were commonly seen as a filter, preventing dust and dirt from reaching the lungs and throat. This was especially valuable during an era in which the filthy city air, seething with miasma, was of great concern. The warmth of beards was thought to ward off toothaches and soothe male vocal cords, an essential benefit for those engaged in frequent public speaking. By the end of the nineteenth century the beard was in sharp decline. Its medical benefits had proven questionable and young men were looking to deviate from their fathers' brand of manhood. The emergence of bodybuilding also played a role, as its most famous practitioners were beardless, instead emphasizing a sporty masculinity through smooth, strong chins and bulging muscles. With the ebb of the beard, those on the fringe who chose to grow their whiskers long were once again displaying a flagrant disregard for social conventions. Their overgrown tresses waved in the wind like dusky flags of resistance. In the decades to come, the beard would return and recede, sometimes signifying rebellion, other times a handsome fad. But its relationship to power remains oppositional, at least in North America and Europe, where politicians have been primarily beardless for over a century.

continued from overleaf —**The bearded crew of HMS** *Folkestone* **hoisting the ship's boat, Freetown, Sierra Leone, circa 1944.**

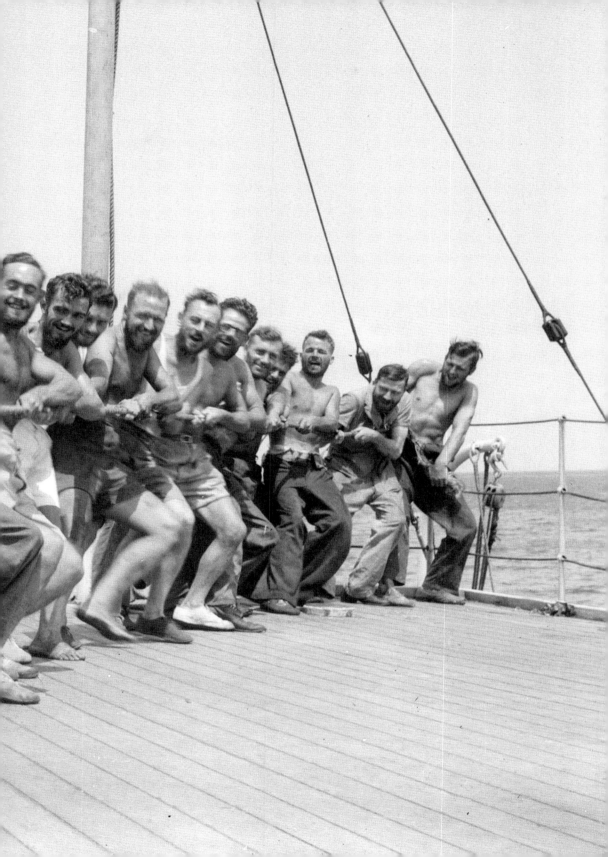

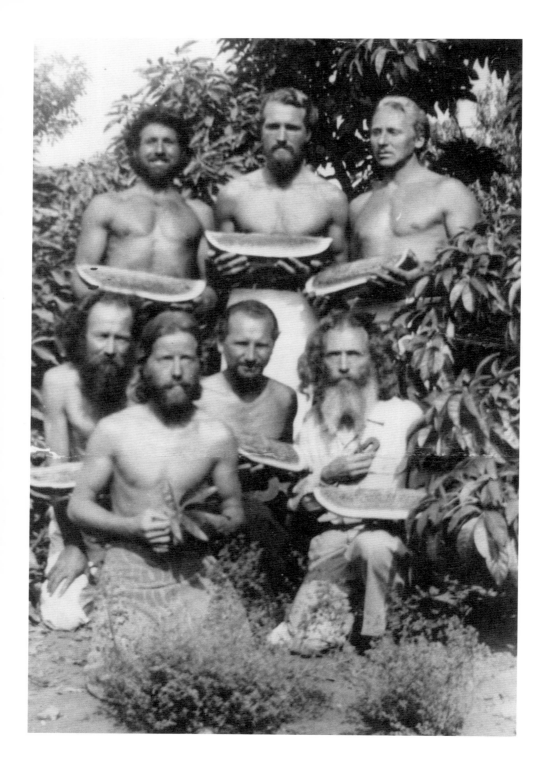

162 The Nature Boys in Topanga Canyon, California, August 1948.

A MILLION BEARDS

A black-and-white photograph from 1948, taken in a canyon near Los Angeles, shows a group of seven mostly bearded and bare-chested men holding long wedges of watermelon. Their faces range from beaming to contemplative, their physiques from ascetic yogi to muscled surfer, and their stance, as though emerging from a bush, invokes their nickname: 'Nature Boys.'

"We all had a common desire to abandon civilization and to live a natural, healthy life," one of them later reflected. Their needs were minimal: sun, water, fresh produce, and some companionship. Another photograph shows them beatifically playing mandolin, guitar, and drum, bare-chested on a sunny sidewalk. These are the only two known photographs showing this loose group of what might be called proto-hippies, or perhaps California Naturemenschen, together.

"We came from different cities, even from different countries," recalled Gypsy Boots, one of the younger members. "At times there were nearly 15 of us, living together in the hills, sleeping in caves and trees." Like their earlier counterparts in central Europe, these Nature Boys foraged for fruit and nuts, sleeping under the stars. In stark contrast to their gentle, pastoral ways, Los Angeles was growing exponentially during and after the Second World War, fanning out in neat grids of suburban housing, two-car garages, and flatly shorn lawns. When the free-wheeling, long-haired men emerged from their rustic hideaways, they must have made quite a spectacle.

Not much is known about the Nature Boys besides hearsay. They make a cameo in Jack Kerouac's *On the Road,* when "an occasional Nature Boy saint in beard and sandals" is glimpsed while passing through late-1940s Los Angeles. But we know they frequented the Richters' Eutropheon café, which drew such types toward it like bees to wild honey. Some of them even found each other there.

One of the Nature Boys, eden ahbez (born George Alexander Aberle in 1908 in Brooklyn), played piano in the Eutropheon's dining room in exchange for meals, sometimes joined by his brethren to form the Nature Boy Trio. His golden wavy hair, full beard, and dreamy, earnest eyes gave him a Christ-like appearance. ahbez, who wrote his chosen name in lowercase because he believed that only the words 'God' and 'Infinity' should be capitalized, claimed to have crossed the country eight times on foot by the time he settled in Los Angeles. He traveled with a sleeping bag, the clothes on his back, and a fruit juicer, scribbling song lyrics along the way. Sometimes ahbez slept in the Richters' backyard among their fruit trees. He also camped in various canyons near the city and for a time made his home in the shadow of the Hollywood sign. He continued this lifestyle with his wife Anna (acquiring a double sleeping bag) and their son named Tatha-Om.

Then there was Maximilian Sikinger, a chiseled German who train-hopped to California in the 1930s, bringing along his homeland's mania for physical culture, nudism, heliotherapy, and natural healing (and also fleeing its rising fascism). One story goes that in San Francisco Sikinger met Gypsy Boots (born Robert Bootzin), and thus found an eager apostle of his Lebensreform philosophies. Boots was already halfway there, raised in a vegetarian household where his Russian mother baked dense black bread and taught her children to forage during Sunday hikes along the railroad tracks. Boots was especially keen to learn more about ways to strengthen the body, having lost his older brother to tuberculosis. Sikinger taught him about fasting and yoga. When the eccentric pair came to Los Angeles, their search for like minds led them to the doorstep of the Eutropheon.

Among the restaurant's most dedicated patrons, conversation likely turned to musings about leaving the city behind for good. The Richters knew of a certain German vegetarian hermit living about 100 miles to the east, in a hut near Palm Springs. Pester must have embodied a shining ideal, a vision of what was possible should city dwellers choose to fully immerse themselves in the natural life.

The sparsely populated desert appealed to the Nature Boys, who often headed out to the arid mountains and their hidden canyons. Tahquitz Canyon was a preferred oasis, a refuge from the heat where a rocky trail led to the rarest of sights: a thin waterfall rushing over massive grey boulders into a pool. It was an ideal place to camp, or even live for several months. Boots later recalled a conversation there with ahbez as they took in the calming beauty of the canyon, where red-tailed hawks carved into the clear sky. "Someday there will be a million beards," ahbez predicted. It took nearly twenty years, but he was right.

If ahbez was in the canyon in the late 1930s, it's possible that he woke one sun-drenched morning to see a wild-haired man treading softly in homemade sandals. It was not a native Cahuilla man nor a sun-blasted homesteader, but a veritable nature boy—rather man, his beard now streaked with white. If ahbez met Pester at Tahquitz, the two certainly would have noticed each other, recognizing kinship.

Their timelines don't line up seamlessly and both contain cryptic blanks. But it has been speculated for years that Pester was a source of inspiration for ahbez's one hit song: "Nature Boy." The original cover of the sheet music, self-published by ahbez in 1946, shows a drawing of a lone man walking in the desert amid prickly cacti, barefoot, bare-chested, and long-haired, with only a small sack thrown over one shoulder. Is it Pester? Is it ahbez himself? Or another, unnamed desert drifter?

HERMITS IN THE CANYONS

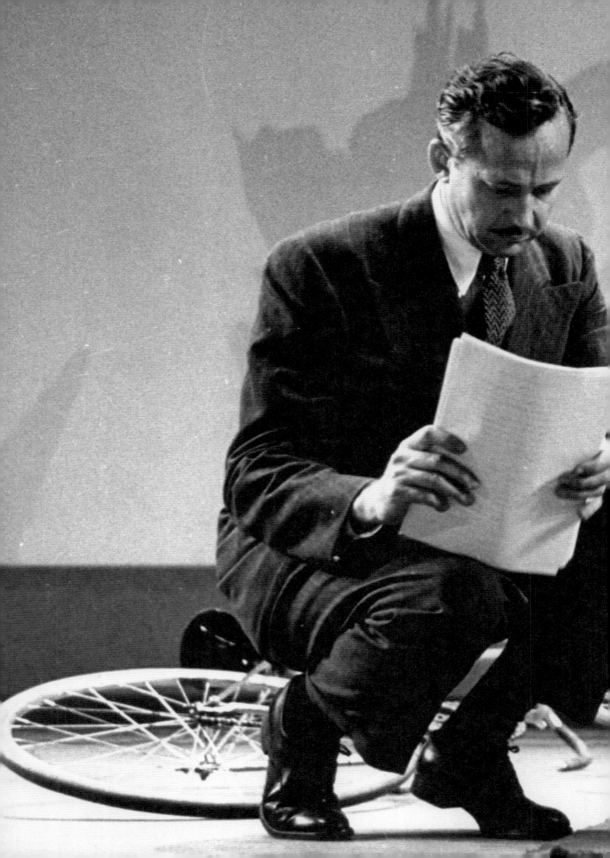

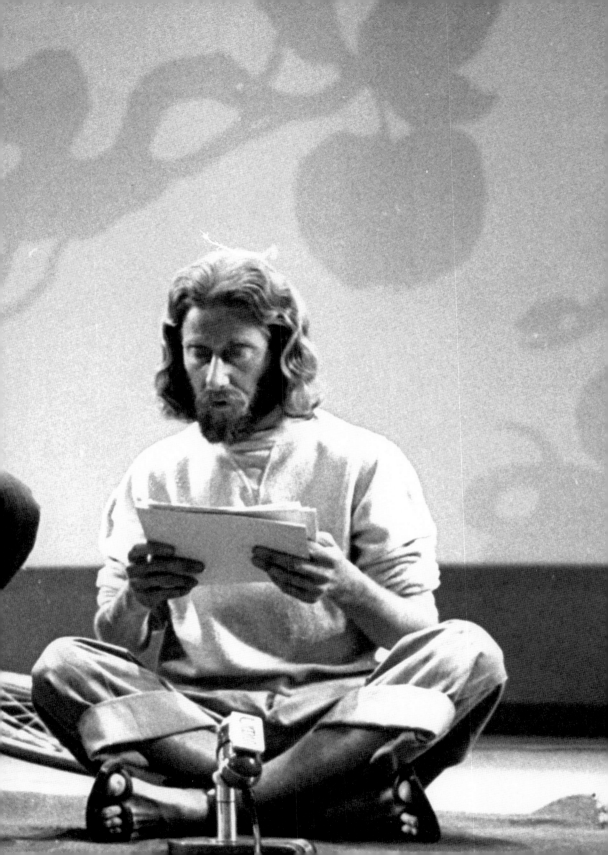

As it turned out, the song itself, and its enigmatic lyrics about "a very strange, enchanted boy / they say he wandered very far, very far, over land and sea" reached millions of listeners. Through a windfall of good fortune, ahbez's song was recorded by Nat King Cole in 1947, rising to the top of the charts and living on as an enduring jazz standard.[7] ahbez was profiled in national magazines and despite becoming suddenly rich, he had no use for the money. In a television interview after his song became famous (he entered the stage in sandals, riding a bicycle), he explained, "All the money in the world will not change my way of life, because all the money in the world could not give me the things I already have. Anna and I have learned that nature, and a simple life, will bring you peace and happiness."

The fates of the Nature Boys eventually diverged. Maximilian Sikinger published a slim diet book called *Classical Nutrition* with a picture of him on the cover kneeling naked on a boulder and reaching up toward the sun. He became an exercise trainer to celebrities and taught at an ashram into his seventies. Boots opened the popular Back to Nature Health Hut restaurant with his wife, Lois, in Hollywood in 1958. It lasted for three years and then he switched to fruit delivery. Eventually he did so in a brightly painted van with "Nuts and Fruits and Gypsy Boots" painted on its side (an echo of Otto Carque's 'health wagon' some fifty years earlier). His antics attracted some health-minded celebrity clientele, and in the early 1960s Boots became a regular guest on a television talk show where he played the madcap nature man, swinging by a rope onto the stage in a loincloth, gulping down freshly squeezed juices and exercising with the host. As a beloved eccentric, Boots shared the stage with many psychedelic bands of the late 1960s, and was considered the 'original hippie,' passing the torch

168

along to a new generation hungry for an alternative way of life.

As for ahbez, he continued living simply and writing music, including *Eden's Island* in 1960, now considered a proto-psychedelic concept album. He was photographed in 1967 holding a wooden flute in a recording studio, sitting next to a young Brian Wilson of the Beach Boys who—following a now-vaunted Los Angeles tradition—had also founded a short-lived health-food store, called the Radiant Radish.[8] Around that same heady year of the Summer of Love, the song "Nature Boy" was given a shimmying, folksy treatment by Jefferson Airplane singer Grace Slick. ahbez's ardent lyrics: "The greatest thing you'll ever learn / is just to love and be loved in return" reached a new audience, reflecting the counterculture's purest idealism.

'Back to nature' was being reborn as 'back to the land,' as an estimated one million people dropped out of society to experiment with rural, communal living. They were driven by a sense that American culture was decaying, similar to the impulse that drove some to flee cities or emigrate from Europe at the turn of the century. It was no longer seen as fresh, wide open, and full of opportunity, but a fruit gone rotten. A new world would be built inside the husk of the old. The anti-establishment dogma, strange diets, and revolutionary badge of long, wild, natural hair returned, spreading more widely than ever before. It all felt radical, groundbreaking, and new.

Even the ravings of Arnold Ehret reappeared. "The beard of man is a secondary sex organ," he had written

---

7. Sleeping near the Hollywood sign had its benefits. The legend goes that ahbez passed his sheet music to Nat King Cole's manager or his valet. With a haunting minor-key melody and folkloric lyrics, "Nature Boy" has been performed and recorded by the likes of Sarah Vaughan, Miles Davis, Ella Fitzgerald, Frank Sinatra, John Coltrane, Sun Ra, David Bowie, and Lady Gaga. It has also graced film soundtracks for the past seventy years.

8. Brian Wilson went through his own obsession with nutrition and fitness, even co-writing a song for the Beach Boys called "Vege-Tables" (1967) with such lyrics as: "I'm gonna keep well my vegetables / Cart off and sell my vegetables / I love you most of all / My favorite vege-table."

HERMITS IN THE CANYONS

in the 1910s. The purified body, he believed, emits electrical "love vibrations" that could be received by "wireless," i.e. hair. When his books were discovered by a new long-haired generation in the 1970s, his publishers replaced Ehret's bearded-but-zealous author photo with a mellowed sketch that gave him a dreamy, prophetic look and a cloud of facial hair. He had found a new era of readers. They were returning to nature, again.

right — eden ahbez playing flute at Gypsy Boots's Health Hut, circa 1958. next spread — Gypsy Boots in Malibu, 1965. The lone bearded man at center, he is holding the April issue of *Esquire* magazine that featured him in an article about relaxed bohemian living called "The Affluent Poor" by Jack Burgess. The subtitle reads: "In Southern California, the very poor are different from you and me — they live better."

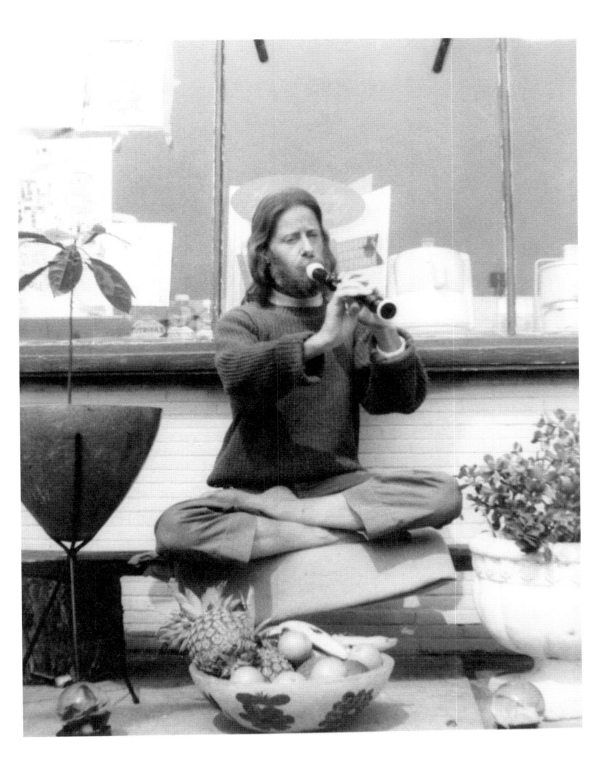

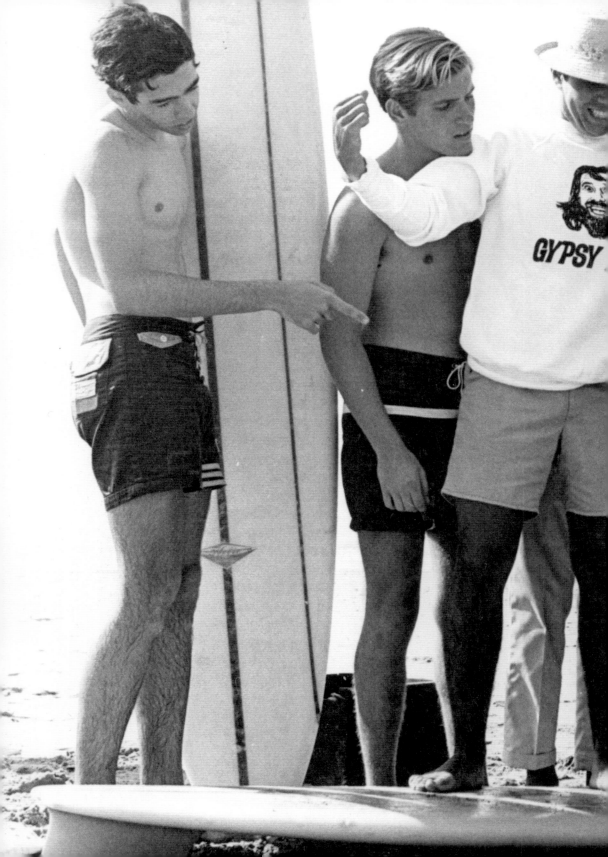

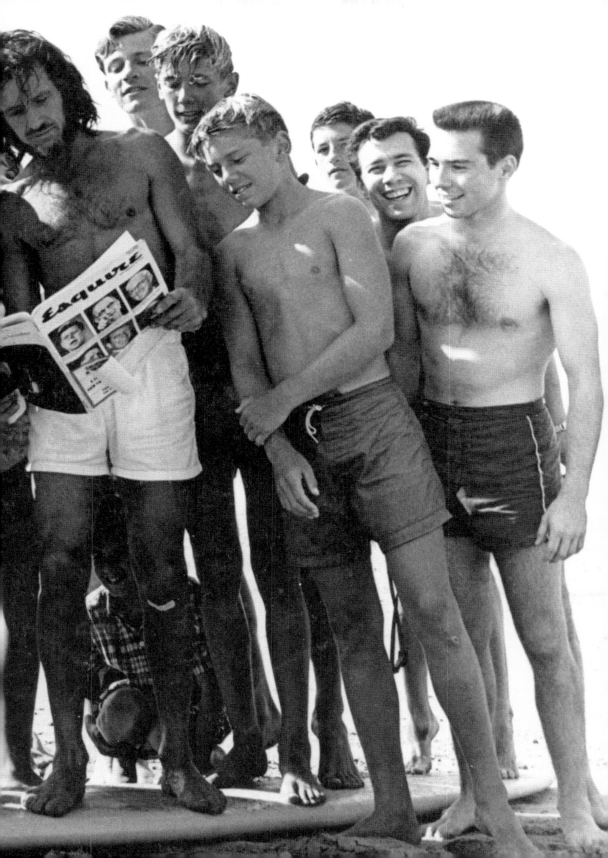

"The lasting, formative influence of the environment on our physiological and psychological health is no less urgent a concern than the debilitating, even lethal contaminants that have been set loose in the life cycles and food chains of the natural world... Such fatigue-prone, nerve-wracking surroundings, seething with stressful impulses and fraught with neurasthenic friction, can literally make us sick."

Richard Neutra, *Nature Near: Late Essays of Richard Neutra*

A fugue between wilderness and industry, or nature and culture, is perennial, as is the belief that the two can be kept separate and in balance. Neutra mounted the headlights of automobiles into the stairwell of Lovell's house of nature-cures to honor the promise of liberation through technological advancement. A couple of decades later the architect lamented: "the infernal combustion engine was winning out against a walkable, healthful, and harmonious world." Neutra was in Los Angeles during the Second World War, when a thick haze, thought be an enemy attack, caused panicking residents to don gas masks. It turned out that the miasma of foul, tear-inducing air was pouring from tailpipes. Modern machines threatened the death of the garden.

Or so it seemed. As the city paved its way up mountains and over orchards, wildness kept hold tenaciously in its seams. Coyotes are still seen trotting suburban streets. Herons glide above the wide concrete channel of the often-forgotten Los Angeles River. Pounds of ripe fruit fall onto sidewalks. And, of course, California's infamous natural catastrophes regularly temper any illusion of human control.

Our maladies, bodily and existential, have evolved since the days of hardbound travelogues hawking healing climates. Maybe it's just that their names, as well as the names of their cures, have changed. Civilization's ills endure, fresh and timeless, and a search for nature, or a more natural lifestyle, persists. It's a false dichotomy but we'll keep trying to separate the strands. Perhaps it isn't nature but an idea of nature, like a talisman, that is so beguiling. On my own brief search for wilderness, as an antidote to staring at a computer screen, I left the city behind to visit Palm Canyon. Where William Pester's shack stood a century ago is a parking lot and souvenir shop that sells chilled bottles of water, T-shirts, and trinkets. But when I walked down the mahogany dirt path to the bottom of the damp canyon, the remote, Edenic allure of the place was still palpable, even spellbinding.

As I wrote and talked about this book I discovered that almost everyone had a related story to tell, even if they were completely disconnected from early Los Angeles or European culture. They lived here, and that was all it took. Some were following the advice of expensive and dubious healers, eating (or more likely not eating) particular foods, or buying into every new 'wellness' regimen. Others were working for greater health equity, trying to bring parks and fresh produce to low-income neighborhoods. (As writer Jennifer Price has noted, some of the city's most polluted neighborhoods contain the factories that manufacture the costly "natural" skincare products sold in wealth-

176

ier, cleaner neighborhoods across town.) One recent transplant from New York breathlessly told me that stepping off the plane here felt like "entering a spa." And I now see that the city's ubiquitous diet and fitness trends are just recycled, like the fashionable new restaurants that mirror their century-old predecessors: one run by a holistic celebrity doctor; another promoting 'living' foods. While I thought I was digging into history, the residues and reverberations of these past health movements are so present that sometimes the eras almost blurred.

Many seekers still come to California in pursuit of an idea—of health, prosperity, and openness. It wasn't until I left this state, where three generations of my family had been born, that its mood and pull became clearer to me. It takes a while for the contradictions of a place to fade into clichés, and longer still to wonder about the roots of those clichés. The mythos of California still circulates, larger than life, capably glossing over intricate realities. It's tethered firmly to this particular land, flourishing in its unique climate, but its origins are stranger, and much older, than we knew.

INDEX

178

BIBLIOGRAPHY

PART 1

Abel, Emily K. *Suffering in the Land of Sunshine: A Los Angeles Illness Narrative*, Rutgers University Press, 2006

Abel, Emily K. *Tuberculosis and the Politics of Exclusion: A History of Public Health and Migration to Los Angeles*, Rutgers University Press, 2007

Ashenburg, Katherine. *The Dirt on Clean: An Unsanitized History*, North Point Press, 2007

Baur, John E. *Health Seekers of Southern California: 1870-1900*, Henry E. Huntington Library and Art Gallery, 2010

Beattie, Andrew. *The Alps: A Cultural History*, Oxford University Press, 2006

Blake, James. "On the Climate and Disease of California," *American Journal of Medical Science*, vol. 24, No. 63, 1852

Chekhov, Anton Pavolovich. *Anton Chekhov's Life and Thought: Selected Letters and Commentary* (edited by Simon Karlinsky, translated by Michael Henry Hein), Northwestern University Press, 1997

Curtis, Ashley (ed.). *O Switzerland!": Travelers' Accounts from 57 BCE to the Present*, Shwabe AG, 2018

Dormandy, Thomas. *The White Death: A History of Tuberculosis*, New York University Press, 2000

Dumke, Glenn. "The Boom of the 1880s In Southern California," *Southern California Quarterly*, vol. 76, No. 1, 1994

Eylers, Eva. "Planning the Nation: The Sanatorium Movement in Germany," *The Journal of Architecture*, vol. 19, No. 5, 667-692, 2014

Harris, Billie and McCready, Linda A. *From Quackery to Quality Assurance: The First Twelve Decades of the Medical Board of California*, Medical Board of California, 1995

Hobday, Richard A., "Sunlight Therapy and Solar Architecture," *Medical History*, vol. 42, 1997

Keers, J. Y. "Two forgotten pioneers. James Carson and George Bodington," *Thorax*, 35, No. 7, 483–489, 1980

Kirchfeld, Friedhelm and Boyle, Wade. *Nature Doctors: Pioneers in Naturopathic Medicine*, NCNM Press, 2005

Logan, Thomas M., "Report of the Permanent Secretary," *First Biennial Report of the State Board of Health of California for the Year 1870*, 1871

McKoon, Hosmer. "Our Glorious Climate," *Land of Sunshine*, June 1894

McWilliams, Carey. *Southern California: An Island on the Land*, Peregrine Smith, 1980

Morrison, Arthur. "Whitechapel," *The Palace Journal*, April 24, 1889

Orgeas, J. *L'hiver à Cannes. Guide descriptif, historique, scientifique, médical et pratique*, Figère et Guiglion, 1889

Praslow, J. *The State of California: A Medico-Geographical Account*, (translated by Frederick Cordes), Newbegin, 1939. (Original edition published in German: Gottingen, 1857)

Remondino, Peter. *The Mediterranean Shores of America: Southern California, its Climatic, Physical, and Meteorological Conditions*, F. A. Davis, 1892

Sontag, Susan. *Illness as Metaphor*, Farrar, Straus, Giroux, 1978

Smith, Peter D. *City: A Guidebook for the Urban Age*, Bloomsbury Press, 2012

Thompson, Kenneth. "The Idea of Longevity in Early California," *Bulletin of the New York Academy of Medicine*, July 1975

Thompson, Kenneth. "Climatotherapy of California" *California Historical Quarterly*, vol. 50, No. 2, 111-130, 1971

Thorsheim, Peter. *Inventing Pollution: Coal, Smoke, and Culture in Britain since 1800*, Ohio University Press, 2006

Trudeau, Edward Livingston. *An Autobiography*, Doubleday, 1916

Vilapana, Cristina. "A Literary Approach to Tuberculosis: Lessons Learned from Anton Chekhov, Franz Kafka, and Katherine Mansfield," *The Journal of Infectious Diseases*, vol. 56, March 2017

Waldier, Donald J. "Border Medicine: Doctors, Disease, and Health-Seekers in L.A.," KCET.org, September 2017

Woloshyn, Tania Anne. *Our Friend, The Sun: Images of Light Therapeutics from the Osler Library Collection, 1901-1944*. Online exhibition, McGill University, 2011

Wood, J. W. *Pasadena: Historical and Personal*, self published, 1917

Zack, Michele. *Southern California Story: Seeking the Better Life in Sierra Madre*, Sierra Madre Historical Preservation Society, 2009

PART 2

Campbell, Margaret. "Strange Bedfellows: Modernism and Tuberculosis," *Imperfect Health: The Medicalization of Architecture*, Giovanna Borasi and Mirko Zardini (eds.), Canadian Centre for Architecture, Lars Muller Publishers, 2012

Campbell, Margaret. "What Tuberculosis did for Modernism: The Influence of a Curative Environment on Modernist Design and Architecture" *Medical History*, vol. 49, No.4, October 2005

Colomina, Beatriz. "X-ray Architecture: Illness as Metaphor," *Positions*, Fall 2008

Colomina, Beatriz. "X-Ray Architecture: An Interview with Beatriz Colomina," *frieze*, No. 18, 2015

Crosse, John. Southern California Architectural History website: https://socalarchhistory.blogspot.com/

Hailey, Charles. "From Sleeping Porch to Sleeping Machine: Inverting Traditions of Fresh Air in North America," *Traditional Dwellings and Settlements Review*, vol. 20, No. 2, Spring 2009

Hines, Thomas S. *Architecture of the Sun: Los Angeles Modernism 1900-1970*, Rizzoli, 2010

Hines, Thomas S. *Richard Neutra and the Search for Modern Architecture: A Biography and History*, University of California Press, 1994

Hobday, Richard. *The Light Revolution: Health, Architecture, and the Sun*, Findhorn Press, 2006

Marmorstein, Gary. "Steel and Slurry: Dr. Philip M. Lovell, Architectural Patron," *The Historical Society of Southern California*, vol. 84, No. 3/4, Fall/Winter 2002

McCoy, Esther. *Vienna to Los Angeles: Two Journeys*, Art + Architecture Press, 1979

McCoy, Esther. "Letters between R. M. Schindler and Richard Neutra, 1914–1924," *Journal of the Society of Architectural Historians*, vol. 33, No. 3, October 1974

Meurs, Paul and van Thoor, Marie-Therese, eds. *Sanatorium Zonnestraal: The History and Restoration of a Modern Monument*, NAi Publishers, 2011

Neutra, Richard. "Aesthetics and the Open Air," *The Studio*, vol. 99, No. 443, February 1930

Neutra, Dione. *Richard Neutra: Promise and Fulfillment*, Southern Illinois University, 1986

Randl, Chad. *Revolving Architecture: A History of Buildings that Rotate, Swivel, and Pivot*, Princeton Architectural Press, 2008

Overy, Paul. *Light, Air, and Openness: Modern Architecture Between the Wars*, Thames & Hudson, 2008

Schrank, Sarah. "Naked Houses: The Architecture of Nudism and Rethinking of the American Suburbs" in Sarah Schrank and Didem Ekici, eds., *Healing Spaces, Modern Architecture, and the Body*, Routledge, 2017

PART 3

Author unknown, *Prosperous California: A Land of Money, Progress and Content*, 1883

Abate, Tom. "State's Little-Known History of Shameful Science / California's Role in Nazis' Goal of 'Purification,'" *San Francisco Gate*, March 2003

Boyle, Wade and Kirchner, Frederick. *Nature Doctors: Pioneers in Naturopathic Medicine*, Medicina Biologica, 1994

Carter, Simon. *Rise and Shine: Sunlight, Technology, and Health*, Berg, 2007

Chidester, Brian. *Bohemian Highways: Art & Culture Abide Then Divide Along the California Coast*, Guardian Stewardship Editions, 2015

Cunningham, Patricia A. *Reforming Women's Fashion, 1850–1920*, Kent State University Press, 2003

Deutsch, Ronald M. *The Nuts among the Berries: An Expose of America's Food Fads*, Ballantine Books, 1961

Deloira, Philip J. *Playing Indian*, Yale University Press, 1999

De Ras, Marion E. P. *Body, Femininity and Nationalism: Girls in the German Youth Movement 1900–1934*, Routledge, 2007

Ekici, Didem. "From Rikli's Light-and-Air Hut to Tessenow's Patenthaus: Korperkultur and the Modern Dwelling in Germany, 1890–1914," *The Journal of Architecture*, vol. 13, No. 4, 379–406, 2008

Freund, Daniel. *American Sunshine: Diseases of Darkness and the Quest for Natural Light*, University of Chicago Press, 2012

Kauffman, Jonathan. *Hippie Food: How Back-to-the-Landers, Longhairs, and Revolutionaries Changed the Way We Eat*, HarperCollins, 2018

Kennedy, Gordon. *Children of the Sun: A Pictorial Anthology from Germany to California, 1883–1949*, Nivaria Press, 1999

Kennedy, Gordon. "Straight-Edge Sexauer," on www.sunfood.net/straight-edge

Kenway, Christopher. "Nudism, Health, and Modernity: The Natural Cure as Proposed by the German Physical Culture Movement 1900–1914," *Nineteenth-Century Prose*, March 1998

Miller, Laura J. *Building Nature's Market: The Business and Politics of Natural Foods*, University of Chicago Press, 2017

Shprintzen, Adam D. *The Vegetarian Crusade: The Rise of an American Reform Movement, 1817–1921*, The University of North Carolina Press, 2013

Ross, Chad. *Naked Germany: Health, Race, and the Nation*, Berg, 2005

Toepfler, Karl. *Empire of Ecstasy: Nudity and Movement in German Body Culture, 1910–1935*, Berkeley: University of California Press, 1997

Waldie, D.J. "How Angelenos Invented the L.A. Summer," *Los Angeles Times*, July 2017

Wild, Peter. *William Pester: The Hermit of Palm Canyon*, Shady Myrick Research Project, 2008

Williams, John Alexander. *Turning to Nature in Germany: Hiking, Nudism, and Conservation, 1900–1940*, Stanford University Press, 2007

Whitman, Walt. *Manly Health and Training: To Teach the Sciences of a Sound and Beautiful Body*, Regan Arts, New York, 2016

Worpole, Ken. *Here Comes the Sun: Architecture and Public Space in European Culture*, Reaktion Books, 2000

NEWSPAPER ARCHIVES

Desert Sun

Los Angeles Times

Los Angeles Herald

San Bernardino Sun

Santa Cruz Sentinel

ARCHIVES

Getty Research Institute

University of California, Los Angeles

Los Angeles Public Library

Palm Springs Historical Society

National University of Natural Medicine

Pasadena Museum of History

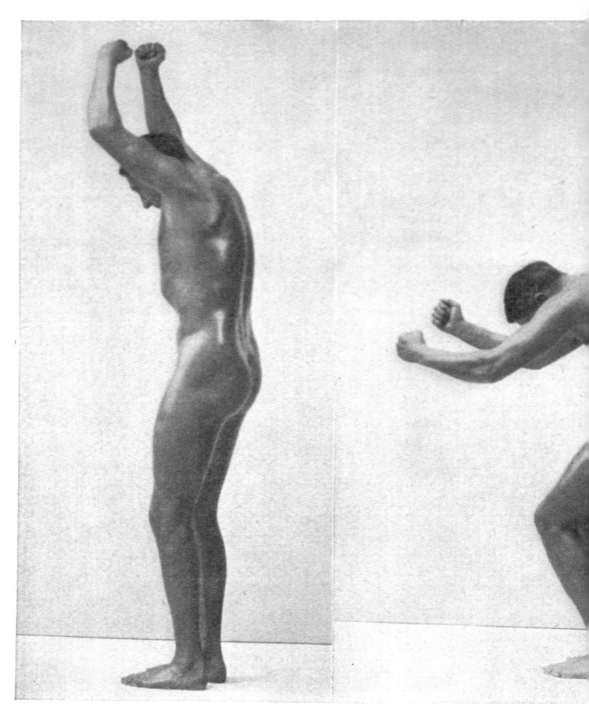

Abb. 90—92. Tiefschwung nach
Ausatmung wäh[...]
Schwung[...]

Beginn der Übung mit voller
Einatmung

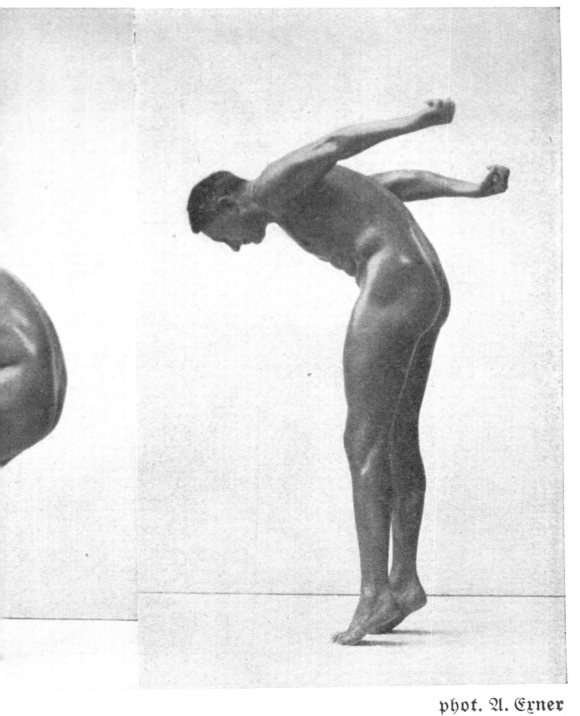

phot. A. Exner

(Surén-Schwunggymnastik)

es   Beendigung des Schwunges und der
                              Ausatmung

IMAGE CREDITS

COVER
The Lovell Health House view from canyon. Photographer Unknown. Courtesy Dion Neutra, Architect © and Richard and Dion Neutra Papers, Department of Special Collections, Charles E. Young Research Library, UCLA

P. 10-11
View of Davos. Sanatorium Davos-Dorf from the side. Edith Södergren's collection Signum: slsa566_282 Photo by Edith Södergran, Swedish Literature Society in Finland

P. 20-21
CA Society for Prevention of Tuberculosis Pamphlet (1908).
Courtesy of the Louise Darling Biomedical Library, Department of Special Collections, University of California Los Angeles

P. 22
Patients sit on balconies of a spa hotel, Davos, Switzerland, circa 1903.
Photo: ullstein bild/ullstein bild via Getty Images

P. 26-27
Patients sit on balconies of a spa hotel, Davos, Switzerland, circa 1903.
Photo: ullstein bild/ullstein bild via Getty Images

P. 31
Sokolowsko Sanatorium. Courtesy of the IN SITU Contemporary Art Foundation and sokolowsko.org

P. 32-34
Ceremony in Memory of Anton Chekhov in Badenweiler 1908. Wikimedia Commons

P. 36
- Man, with blanket over lap, seated in front of a small building in a tuberculosis camp. Ottawa, Illinois, circa 1908. Photo by George Grantham Bain, Library of Congress
- Tuberculosis hospital and sanatorium construction plan, circa 1911. Wikimedia Commons
- The Little Red Cottage, Adirondack Cottage Sanitarium (now Trudeau Sanatorium), Saranac Lake, New York. From *An autobiography* by Edward Livingston Trudeau, 1848-1915

P. 40
- Pages from the *Journal of The Outdoor Life*, published at the Adirondack Cottage Sanitarium in Saranac Lake, New York, 1905
- Men lounge in chairs (before the 'cure chair' was designed) on deck. Adirondack Cottage Sanitarium, Saranac Lake, New York, circa 1905. Courtesy of the Adirondack Experience - The Museum on Blue Mountain Lake

P. 41
Pages from the Journal of *The Outdoor Life*, published at the Adirondack Cottage Sanitarium in Saranac Lake, New York, 1905

P. 42
Panoramic view of the Barlow Sanatorium in Elysian Park, Los Angeles, California, circa 1915. Wikimedia Commons

P. 46-47
Pages from The Land of Sunshine, 1894-1895

P. 51
- Pottenger Sanatorium, Monrovia, California, circa 1923. Courtesy of the California History Room, California State Library, Sacramento, California
- Dr. F. M. Pottenger, Sr. at his sanatorium, circa 1903. Courtesy of the Monrovia Historical Society

P. 52-55
Boys sunbathing. Security Pacific National Bank Collection, Los Angeles Public Library

P. 125
Photographer unknown. Bellinzona, Archivio di Stato del Cantone Ticino,
Archivio Fondazione Monte Verità, Fondo Harald Szeemann.

P. 126
Portrait of August Engelhardt. Courtesy of Christian Kracht

P. 130-131
George Grantham Bain Collection, Library of Congress, Prints & Photographs Division,
[LC-DIG-ggbain-01504]

P. 135
Mensendieck school, Oslo. Wikimedia Commons, from the National Library of Norway

P. 139
Demonstration of exercises from Hans Surén's *Atemgymnastik*, 1929

P. 140-143
Display of "Eugenics in New Germany" in Pasadena, California, circa 1934.
Courtesy of the Deutsches Hygiene-Museum

P. 144
View of Downtown Los Angeles Restaurant. Security Pacific National Bank Collection,
Los Angeles Public Library

P. 152
– Granola Advertisement, Wikimedia Commons
– Advertisement for the Nature Cure Supply Centre, run by Benedict Lust.
Courtesy of the Rare Books Archive and Library of National University of Natural Medicine.
Benedict Lust archival collection, 1900–1923
– Advertisements for the Eutropheon and The Vegetarian restaurants

P. 156
Portrait of Arnold Ehret. From his book *Rational Fasting*

P. 158-161
HMS Folkestone's bearded crew. March 1944, Freetown, Sierra Leone.
Courtesy of the Imperial War Museum © IWM (A 22949)

P. 162
Nature Boys, Topanga Canyon, August 1948. Photographer Unknown. Estate of Gypsy Boots.
Thanks to Gordon Kennedy

P. 166-167
eden ahbez on We The People TV series, circa 1948. Photo by Peter Stackpole.
The LIFE Picture Collection/Getty Images

P. 171
eden ahbez at Gypsy Boots's Health Hut, circa 1958. Estate of Gypsy Boots.
Thanks to Gordon Kennedy

P. 172-173
Gypsy Boots in Malibu. Estate of Gypsy Boots. Thanks to Gordon Kennedy

P. 186-187
Demonstration of exercises from Hans Surén's *Atemgymnastik*, 1929

IMAGE CREDITS

AUTHOR ACKNOWLEDGEMENTS

I would like to thank the wonderful team of collaborators who made this book possible, foremost my intrepid publishers, Kingston and Pascale, for their enthusiasm, vision, and extraordinary trust; my editor Ananda for descending into the trenches with me and deftly lighting the way; Capucine for her stunning design; and Andrew, Gregor, and Rich for expertly combing through facts and language, making both more precise. I salute the librarians and archivists of Southern California for generously helping me track down materials and safeguarding these histories. To my friends and family, your excitement and support has been sustaining, from the first mention to the finish line. Special acknowledgements to my father, who introduced me to the song "Nature Boy" as a child and my mother, who keeps on planting trees. Lastly, my ardent thanks to Robert Amesbury, my first reader, who gave wise feedback and steadfast optimism every step of the way, and to our daughter Sonya for her daily wonder and joy.

AUTHOR
Lyra Kilston

EDITING
Ananda Pellerin

SUB-EDITING
Gregor Shepherd

FACT-CHECKING
Andrew St. Maurice

PROOFREADING
Helius

INDEXING
Annette Musker

DESIGN
Capucine Labarthe

PUBLISHED BY
Atelier Éditions
Los Angeles, California
London, United Kingdom
www.atelier-editions.com

Edition of 3000
Printed in Spain
on 100% ecological paper
from sustainable forests

ISBN # 978-0-9975935-8-7